# A Caregiver's GUIDE

## A HANDBOOK ABOUT END-OF-LIFE CARE

*Karen Macmillan Jacquie Peden*

*Jane Hopkinson Dennie Hycha*

**PUBLISHED BY**

The Military and Hospitaller Order
of St. Lazarus of Jerusalem

**IN ASSOCIATION WITH**

The Canadian Hospice Palliative Care Association

A handbook about end-of-life care

REVISED 2014

Published by
The Military and Hospitaller Order of St. Lazarus of Jerusalem
in assocation with Canadian Hospice Palliative Care Association



1435 Sandford Fleming Avenue, Suite 100, Ottawa, ON K1G 3H3
(613) 746-5280 website: www.stlazarus.ca • email: *chancery@stlazarus.ca*



Library and Archives Canada Cataloguing in Publication Data:

*A Caregiver's Guide: a Handbook About End-of-Life Care*/Macmillan, Karen ... [et al.

Co-published by Canadian Hospice Palliative Care Association. Includes bibliographic references and index.

ISBN: 0-9686700-1-6

1. Terminally ill-Home care-Handbooks, manuals, etc. 2. Palliative treatment-Handbooks, manuals, etc. I. Macmillan, Karen II. Hospitallers of St. Lazarus of Jerusalem. III. Canadian Hospice Palliative Care Association.

R726.8.C371 2004 649.8 C2004-904456-7

The Canadian Hospice Palliative Care Association
Annex D, Saint Vincent Hospital, 60 Cambridge Street North
Ottawa, Ontario K1R 7A5
Phone: (613) 241-3663, 1-800-668-2785

*A Caregiver's Guide* will be provided to family caregivers across Canada by their local hospices, palliative care programs or provincial palliative care and hospice associations which may acquire it at a nominal cost from the Canadian Hospice Palliative Care Association. Others may purchase this book from the Canadian Hospice Palliative Care Association or the Order of St. Lazarus.

Cover Design by Joni Millar, Tilt Creative
Original design, layout and illustrations by Robert Weidemann
Printed and bound in Canada by Marquis Book Printing

# DEDICATION

■

*A Caregiver's Guide is dedicated to*

*those Canadians caring for and about*

*their friends and loved ones*

*on their final journey.*

*We hope this book will provide some*

*extra support and help to them.*

" Be near me when my light is low"

*In Memoriam*
*Alfred, Lord Tennyson*

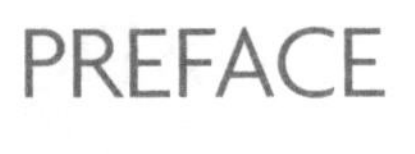


■

Supporting a loved one who is dealing with a terminal illness is an incredibly difficult situation. However, no one should ever have to endure the physical and emotional suffering brought on by a terminal illness on their own, and family often becomes a very important part of coping.

A growing number of Canadians are expressing a preference for care in their own home in familiar and comfortable surroundings. This means that the role of family caregiver is growing and taking on a wider range of tasks and responsibilities. Their willingness to provide support at home makes it possible for many Canadians to be cared for in the setting of their choice.

Too often there is little support or understanding of the important role the informal caregiver provides. Usually it is a patient's closest family member, such as a spouse or adult child, who is asked to provide emotional and personal support. In some cases, they may be thrust into a role they feel unprepared for. In other cases, they may be asked to make critical decisions about the care of their loved one. There is no doubt that family caregivers suffer along with the patient, but their own needs are often overlooked.

That is why *A Caregiver's Guide* is such a useful resource. It provides guidance and assistance and addresses the many fears and uncertainties about terminal illness and caregiving in clear and simple terms. Further, it focusses on the physical, emotional, and spiritual needs of patients and their families.

Our government has supported several initiatives to help with the delivery of palliative care in a variety of settings, and has aided in the training of front-line healthcare providers in palliative care. As our society becomes increasingly aware of the importance of family caregiving towards the end of life, and the role of family caregivers continues to evolve, it is important to ensure that supports such as this guide are available to assist them on this difficult journey.

*Honourable Rona Ambrose PC, MP,*
*Minister of Health,*
*Government of Canada*

# THE DEVELOPMENT OF *A CAREGIVER'S GUIDE*

■

This 2013 revised national edition of *A Caregiver's Guide: a Handbook About End-of-Life Care* was developed by the Military and Hospitaller Order of St. Lazarus and the Canadian Hospice Palliative Care Association. The history of its origin and subsequent editions can be found in Appendix IX (page 165).

This national edition was reviewed by palliative care professionals from across Canada.

## AUTHORS AND REVIEWERS

### Original Publication Committee

Dennie Hycha RN, MN
Robert W. Clarke CD, GCLJ, MCFP (Hon)
Carleen Brenneis RN, MHSA
Jane Hopkinson BN, MN
Karen Macmillan RN, BScN,
Jacquie Peden RN, MN
Edna McHutchion PhD,
Pam Berry Otfinowski RN, BA, BScN
Norman Sande BEd, MEd, KCLJ

## 2013 REVIEW COMMITTEE

Requests for general feedback from key people in every province were sent out, and we are extremely grateful for their input and the conversations that took place. Moreover, a cross section of specific hospice palliative care professionals from across the country kindly agreed to review chapters.

## NATIONAL LEADS THIRD REVIEW EDITION:

### Project Oversight

Robert W. Clarke, Project Director,
The Order of St. Lazarus

Sharon Baxter, Executive Director,
Canadian Hospice Palliative Care Association

**Project Coordination**

Laurie Anne O'Brien,
President, Canadian Hospice Palliative Care Association

**Project Assistant**

Julia Ehrhardt, Canadian Hospice Palliative Care Association

## CHAPTER REVIEWERS:

Laurie Anne O'Brien, RN BN CHPCN(C),
Independent Consultant/Educator, Palliative and End of Life Care

Wendy Wainwright BSW, Med
Manager, Psychosocial Services, Victoria Hospice Society, Victoria, BC

Maryse Bouvette RN, BScN, MEd, CON(C), CHPCN(C)
Coordinator of the Palliative Pain and Symptom Management Consultation Service, Palliative Care Program
Bruyère Continuing Care, 43 Bruyère Street, Ottawa, ON

Carmel Collins RN BN NP-PHC CHPCN(C)
Nurse Practitioner, Regional Palliative Care Leadership Team, Eastern Health St. John's, NL

Jennifer Forward MClSc OT
Occupational Therapist, Eastern Health, Carbonear, NL

Patricia A. McQuinn, RN, BSc Mj; MScA(Nursing), CHPCN(C)
Clinical Nurse Specialist, Palliative
Extra-Mural Driscoll, Horizon Health Network, Moncton, NB

Dr. Heather Mohan Van Heerden PhD, RCC, MTA
Executive Director/Program Coordinator: Camp Kerry Society (Burnaby, BC), Bereavement Coordinator/Music Therapist, Delta Hospice Society (Delta, BC), Former family caregiver

# PLANNING AHEAD: HAVING THE CONVERSATION

■

Many of us shy away from having conversations with loved ones about what kind of medical and personal care we would want, especially in the event of a life-threatening or progressive illness. Difficult as it may be, it is important for all of us to start the conversation, and start it early. We need to share our health and personal care wishes with each other at various times of our lives, including the final stage. One way to begin this process is to explore and engage in the conversation by using Advance Care Planning (ACP) resources as a guide.

Advance Care Planning is a process of reflection and communication. It helps us let others know our future health and personal care preferences, especially if we later become incapacitated and unable to speak for ourselves. Having these invaluable conversations early ensures a degree of trust and confidence in our wishes, knowing that they will be considered in later stages of life. Most family members have indicated that these conversations, along with the creation of reference documents, significantly reduce the stress and burden on caregivers and other family members.

During creation of an Advance Care Plan, a person (sometimes called a Substitute Decision Maker) is often named to speak for you if you are unable to do so. ACP may also involve conversations with family members, healthcare providers, and financial and legal professionals.

Many provinces and territories have specific resources that relate to their own ACP legislation. A number have forms that can be used for documenting your substitute decision maker and your wishes. Please visit your region's website for further details.

Moreover, the Advance Care Planning website provides people with the tools and resources needed to effectively engage in the process of documenting end-of-life wishes. Please visit *advancecareplanning.ca* for details.

# CONSIDERING BECOMING A CAREGIVER

■

The caregiving experience is unique and special for everyone. In order to be prepared for this new role, it is important to reflect early on a number of questions: What does being a caregiver mean for you and your loved one? What help do you hope to provide? What help are you able to provide? What support and training would be beneficial? It is also worthwhile to clarify expectations at the beginning of your caregiving journey, as they can be much harder to alter as your loved one's illness progresses and your role has already been assumed.

Your loved one may say they want to die at home. This is a big decision and commitment for everyone involved. While the first instinct of many caregivers is to automatically say yes, it is important to make a measured decision. Take into account your own needs, those of your loved ones and the advice of the healthcare team. In so doing, you will be more prepared as your loved one's illness progress and their care needs evolve. Taking the time to explore these issues will give you an accurate picture of the time commitment involved, the energy required, and the extra supports you will need to manage the emotional, physical and financial aspects of caregiving. This guide will help you organize a present and future plan of care that can help to reduce stress. When you plan for care, especially at home, be sure to explore *A Caregiver's Guide* ahead of time.

Also, consider the following questions, which have been provided by previous family caregivers:

- Do you have all the necessary information from a hospital and/or home care team about ongoing physical and practical needs that will help you to provide your loved one's total care at home?
- Do you feel you can meet care needs on a short and/or long-term basis?
- Have you considered the impact of your new role on all of your relationships, not just with the loved one who is receiving care?
- What about your social life, coping strategies, and your physical and emotional health?
- How might this role affect your work?
- Would your work grant you a leave of absence? Have you considered applying for the Compassionate Care Benefit through Service Canada? (See Appendix VII Compassionate Care Program.)
- Have you developed contingency plans that would allow for extra home care, admittance to a hospice or palliative care program should the need arise?

# TABLE OF CONTENTS

INTRODUCTION

Hospice Palliative Care....3
Contact Names and Numbers....4

1 WHEN A PROGRESSIVE LIFE-THREATENING ILLNESS IS DIAGNOSED

Coming to Terms with What is Happening....8
Caring for Yourself - The Caregiver....11
Support Networks....16
Communication with Others....18
Spiritual Needs....23
Adapting Your Home....25

2 GIVING PHYSICAL CARE

Infection Control (Universal Precautions)....28
Bathing....30
Mouth Care....33
Positioning Someone in Bed....35
Helping Someone Move Up in Bed....38
Making a Bed....40
Helping with Moving About....43
Moving Someone From Bed to Chair....45
Walking....46
Toileting....48
Food and Fluid Changes....51
Giving Help with Eating....54
Nutritional Supplement Recipes....58
Liquid Feedings....59
Medications....60

3 CARE OF PHYSICAL PROBLEMS

Pain....70
Managing Pain with Medications....72
Possible Side Effects or Complications of Opioids....75
Other Ways to Manage Pain Relief....78
Skin Problems....79

Mouth Problems ... 82
Bowel and Bladder Problems ... 86
Shortness of Breath (Dyspnea) ... 91
Nausea and Vomiting ... 94
Trouble Sleeping (Insomnia) ... 96
Swelling (Edema) ... 97
Loss of Strength ... 98
Confusion ... 99
Complementary Care ... 101

4 AS LIFE ENDS

Planning ... 110
A Move to Hospice, Palliative Care, Long Term Care or Hospital ... 113
Last Days of Life ... 114
Signs That Death is Approaching ... 116
When Death Occurs ... 117
Grief ... 125
Final Thoughts ... 131

5 BOOKS AND OTHER RESOURCES THAT MAY BE HELPFUL

Written Materials ... 134
Books to Help Grieving Children ... 138
Internet Resources ... 139
References Used in Preparation of This Book ... 142
Appendix I Financial Aid ... 146
Appendix II Legal Affairs ... 149
Appendix III Home Medication Schedule ... 151
Appendix IV Symptom Assessment Scale ... 152
Appendix V Breakthrough Medication Chart ... 153
Appendix VI Further Medical, Legal and Financial Provincial Contacts ... 154
Appendix VII Compassionate Care Program ... 162
Appendix VIII Planning Ahead For the Funeral ... 163
Appendix IX History of *A Caregiver's Guide* ... 165
Appendix X The Military and Hospitaller Order of St. Lazarus of Jerusalem .. 168
Appendix XI Canadian Hospice Palliative Care Association ... 173
Index ... 176
Notes for you and your nurse ... 180
We'd Like Your Help ... 182

# INTRODUCTION

# BEING A CAREGIVER

■

As you begin to take care of a loved one with a progressive illness, you are facing what many describe as one of the most profoundly rewarding, yet at times overwhelming, personal experiences of your life. It will not be easy. It will be especially difficult to understand the ongoing progression of your loved one's illness, which will emotionally and physically change your family member.

But who is a caregiver? A caregiver can be a family member, a friend or a group of people who are available to provide care for a loved one at home. A caregiver should take some time to consider many factors, including his or her physical and emotional health ability and the time required to provide care. If time off work is required, the federal government now offers a Compassionate Care Benefit program for those providing care or support to a gravely ill family member. (See Appendix VII Compassionate Care Program.)

As a caregiver, you are encouraged to reach out to others and allow them to help make sure you do not feel alone. Find out what supports and resources are in your area, such as caregiver networks, support groups and home health care teams. Your health care team may consist of the family doctor, home care nurse, other health care workers, a pastor or spiritual adviser, volunteers, family members, and friends. With a team approach the physical, emotional, psychological and spiritual needs of not only your loved one, but also you and your family, can be met. Share your concerns or cultural and spiritual practices with your team. Your team can help you and your loved one cope with stages of the illness and the dying process, while striving to make this final journey as comfortable as possible.

Even when you have committed yourself to this role, you will need to take breaks from the caregiving. This is called self-care. You may need to take breaks for a few minutes to go for a walk, read a book, or talk to a friend. Respite care can help if you feel you need a longer break. Always remember that it is okay to review and change your mind about your decision to be a caregiver at any time.

> ***"Aim to do the best you can with what you have for the time you have."***
>
> *– Author unknown*

Care at the final stages of life is called palliative care or hospice care. To better understand its meaning, the following definition is given through the Canadian Hospice Palliative Care Norms of Practice.

# HOSPICE PALLIATIVE CARE

■

Hospice palliative care aims to relieve suffering and improve the quality of living and dying.

Hospice palliative care strives to help patients and families:
- address physical, psychological, social, spiritual and practical issues, and their associated expectations, needs, hopes and fears.
- prepare for life closure and the dying process.
- cope with loss and grief during the illness and bereavement.

Hospice palliative care aims to:
- treat all active issues.
- prevent new issues from occurring.
- promote opportunities for meaningful and valuable experiences, personal and spiritual growth, and self-actualization.

Hospice palliative care is appropriate for any patient and/or family living with, or at risk of developing, a life-threatening illness due to any diagnosis, with any prognosis, regardless of age, and at any time they have unmet expectations and/or needs, and are prepared to accept care.

Hospice palliative care may complement and enhance disease-modifying therapy or it may become the total focus of care.

Hospice palliative care is most effectively delivered by an interdisciplinary team of healthcare providers who are both knowledgeable and skilled in all aspects of the caring process related to their discipline of practice. These providers are typically trained by schools or organizations that are governed by educational standards. Once licensed, providers are accountable to standards of professional conduct that are set by licensing bodies and/or professional associations.

Definition from *A Model to Guide Hospice Palliative Care*

Bear some points about the use of this handbook in mind:

- Medical words that might not be understood have been explained. The pages where these explanations can be read are indicated in the Index.
- Throughout the book, suggestions have been made for brand name products available for dealing with particular problems. This list is by no means complete and many similar products work just as well. Ask your pharmacist, doctor or health care nurse for advice. Any mention of specific brands does not mean the developers of this guide endorse this product.

# CONTACT NAMES AND NUMBERS

■

Throughout the guide, under the heading 'Important Points,' it has been suggested that you call or ask for help about specific things. The information about who to call has not been included because each person's needs, as well as contact information in your area, may be different. To get in touch with the right people, you often need to call your home care nurse. Ask a member of your health care team to help identify who you should call for a particular concern. On the next page, you will find a chart that you can fill in to compile a list of important contacts. You might find it helpful to photocopy this page and keep it in a prominent place, such as near the phone or on your fridge. There are also blank pages at the end of the book where you can make notes about your specific needs and people who can help you.

| NAME | NUMBER |
| --- | --- |
| Family doctor | Home care coordinator |
| | |
| Home care nurse (CLSC in Quebec) | Physiotherapist |
| | |
| Occupational therapist | Social worker |
| | |
| Support worker/Homemaker | Volunteer |
| | |
| Pastor or spiritual advisor | Pharmacist |
| | |
| Respiratory therapist | Respiratory equipment vendor |
| | |
| Dietitian | Family and friends |
| | |

## OTHER CONTACTS

| | |
| --- | --- |
| | |
| | |
| | |
| | |
| | |

## OTHER CONTACTS

| | |
|---|---|
| | |
| | |
| | |
| | |
| | |
| | |
| | |
| | |
| | |
| | |
| | |
| | |
| | |
| | |

CHAPTER

1

# WHEN A PROGRESSIVE LIFE-THREATENING ILLNESS IS DIAGNOSED

# COMING TO TERMS WITH WHAT IS HAPPENING

■

When someone very close to you has been told they have a progressive life-threatening illness, it is a life-changing event for everyone. It can take a long or short time and much effort to come to terms with what is happening. For everyone involved, there will be a very normal sense of shock, change, loss, uncertainty, anxiety, fear and hope.

During this time, as a caregiver you may find that:
- time stands still.
- priorities change.
- life and death take on new meanings.
- things you previously took for granted are changed forever.
- your hopes for the future now have to shift and change.
- life may even lose its present purpose and meaning.

## WHAT YOU MAY EXPECT

The knowledge that death is not as far away can color all aspects of daily living.
- Shock, numbness, disbelief, panic, helplessness and hopelessness are common.
- Many past losses and changes as well as current and future ones are now to be considered. These can include family roles, control over life events, body image, sexual feelings, financial changes, future hopes and dreams.
- Increased fears can occur relating to body changes, the final days, death, possible uncontrollable symptoms, and overall pain and suffering.
- Mixed and changing emotions can feel like a roller-coaster ride.
- At times, you may deny what is happening. At other moments, the reality of what you are feeling and understanding may seem too much to bear.
- Sometimes you may think that others do not seem to care or understand as much as you do.
- Anger, sadness, guilt and blame can seem overwhelming.
- You may have periods of questioning. "Why did this happen to us?"

These feelings may go on for quite some time or change from day to day, and hour to hour. As you grieve each new change and loss as the illness progresses, it may seem as if you are in a dream from which you hope you will soon wake.

## REMEMBER:

All these reactions are normal.

- Each person's response to difficult news, change, loss and grief is very personal and must unfold in its own time and in its own way.
- While there may be no set ways or quick fixes to help you through, please know that there are still people and things that may help.

## WHAT MAY HELP YOU AND YOUR LOVED ONE

- Take your cues from how your loved one is feeling, and acknowledge your feelings as well. Keeping a daily journal may help you.
- Be as open and truthful as you can, especially when you or your loved one is doing poorly. Everyone, whether sick or well, needs to be treated with caring respect, understanding and honesty.
- Respect the privacy of the sick person and allow them as much control as possible when making decisions about their care and activities.
- Go easy on giving advice. Be prepared and open to having it ignored and rejected at times.
- Share hopes, thoughts and feelings. It can provide comfort to you both, and build a better understanding and meaning of what is important now and how to best support one another.
- Enjoy the good days and make the best of your times together.
- Reminisce about your life together – the good and the not so good.
- Include your loved one in family activities whenever possible.
- Spend time together talking, listening to music, watching television, playing cards or games. Share your thoughts and feelings, laughter and tears.
- Try to resolve any conflicts or unfinished business that you may have. If this is difficult, perhaps a third person can help.
- Help your loved one put their affairs in order. Having an advanced care plan, completing or updating the will, settling the estate, sharing financial documents, accounts, investments, credit cards, mortgage information and the location of all important documents can help you both to prepare. Seek to understand more fully about what you may need to know about any financial or other help (see Appendix I *Financial Aid*, page 146).
- Take care of yourself physically and emotionally. Eat healthy foods and try to exercise and relax. Reach out and talk about your feelings and concerns with someone you trust and who understands you and your situation. This might be a family member, friend, counsellor or religious advisor.
- Keep up some important family routines and let the others go for a while.

- Know and accept your limits. You cannot provide all the answers, solve all the problems or provide all the care. Accept help from others who want to be involved.

## WHAT YOU MIGHT EXPECT AS YOUR LOVED ONE'S ILLNESS PROGRESSES

Your loved one may experience:

- changing emotions, hopes and needs.
- increasing fear, yearning, anxiety, edginess, irritability and sadness.
- feelings such as confusion, powerlessness and uncertainty about what to do.
- mood swings between periods of denial and acceptance, hopefulness and hopelessness.
- withdrawal from normal life activities and people due to increased tiredness.
- changing physical appearance that causes reluctance to be with others.
- concerns about increasing care needs and being a burden.

You may:

- become exhausted, distracted and worry about how you are coping now and how you are going to cope in the future.
- be increasingly aware of dying, death and your own mortality.

### IMPORTANT POINTS

*Do not tell a sad person to "cheer up" as this can create further anxiety and distance.*

*Ask your care team for help if:*

- *fear, anxiety, sadness or depression are severe, or go on for several days, or the person expresses thoughts of suicide.*
- *the person suddenly refuses to eat, cannot sleep or takes no interest in daily activities. Remember these are normal things that can usually happen over a period of time as the illness progresses.*
- *feelings of guilt, worthlessness and hopelessness are strong.*
- *the person shows new symptoms of anxiety, complaining of being unable to breathe, is sweating or is very restless.*
- *you as caregiver are tired, feel overwhelmed and need help or relief.*

# CARING FOR YOURSELF - THE CAREGIVER

■

Caring for a loved one who has a progressive illness can be rewarding, but it can also be physically and emotionally challenging and draining. It is often difficult to predict how long you will be providing care. You must make sure that you take care of yourself as well. By taking care of yourself you will be better able to take care of your loved one.

## WHAT YOU CAN DO TO CARE FOR YOURSELF

When caring for others, it is easy to put off or forget to care for yourself. You need to attend to your basic needs such as eating well, getting enough rest, exercising and seeking out emotional support. Look for ways to ease your workload and share tasks among family and friends. Find out what services are available in your community and use them. Go to professionals for help with your health concerns, counseling, and financial or legal needs. You need to be realistic and know your limitations on what you feel you can take on and handle, as well as what is available to you for help.

To keep yourself as healthy as possible:

- Proper meals are important. You need to eat on a regular schedule even when you are feeling too tired or too busy.
- Prepare more meal portions when you or others cook so you have extra healthy meals in the freezer.
- Stock up on healthy snacks such as fruit, cheese, yogurt, peanut butter, and whole grain crackers for times when you are very busy and still need to eat.
- Make time for regular exercise such as walking, swimming, stationary or regular bicycling.
- Keep up with your regular dental and medical appointments.
- Try planning your sleep around your loved one's sleep schedule.
- If you have a career or part-time job, consider taking a leave of absence and applying for compassionate care benefits (see Appendix VII Compassionate Care Program, page 162).

## Coping skills

Caring for someone with a progressive illness, while a rewarding and a special gift to your loved one, can take its toll on you mentally and physically. It is normal to feel despair and sadness or anger and frustration at your situation, but the way you cope with and manage those feelings will make a big difference. Always remember to:

- Call on family or friends to help you when the load seems too heavy. They can assist with tasks such as making meals, and other forms of respite care.
- Get help with household chores if needed by hiring someone to do heavy work such as laundry and vacuuming. If you have a home care nurse, ask if this type of support is available in your community.
- Let go of any guilt you may feel by taking a break when you need it, and strive to focus on something other than illness and caregiving.
- Remember that others are also trying to cope in their own way. Try to see things from their perspective when tense situations arise.
- Break down big problems into a smaller size by working through them one step at a time.
- Set realistic goals for yourself and do what you are able to do.
- Set aside special time for others in your life. Consider scheduling it into your day or week.

## Managing your emotions

Most people find 114that they have conflicting and changing emotions at this time. You may feel up one day and down the next. You may be sad and angry at the same time. You may feel increased inner strength and resolve one day, and hopeless and helpless the next. Feeling sad, angry, afraid, frustrated, and anxious are normal in times of stress. You may be grieving the anticipated death and loss of your loved one, and angry that they are going to die. Remember that there is no right way to feel at this time.

- Find healthy ways to relieve tension and blow off steam through vigorous exercise, pounding a pillow, or sitting alone in a private space such as your car and just yelling.
- If you feel resentment, get it off your chest. If you need a sounding board, talk to a friend, family member, or professional.
- Find out if your community has a support group where you can talk with others who are in your position and understand your feelings. Your home care nurse or local health care authority can direct you to groups in your region.

- If you are having emotional difficulty caring for your loved one because of a history of abuse, addiction or conflict, talk to someone.
- Keep up with activities that are comforting and meaningful to you. These may include gardening, crafts, reading, community meetings or being with friends and family.
- It is good to share humour and smiles, laugh and cry without feeling guilty. It is a healthy way to release tension and focus on living your best each day.
- Try to stay away from people who make you angry or situations you find frustrating.
- Write about your thoughts, feelings and experiences in a journal.
- Practice deep breathing and relaxation techniques.
- Give yourself a pat on the back for whatever you are able to do to help.

### Respite care

Respite means taking a break from the responsibilities of being a caregiver, whether through getting extra help in your home or seeking out a respite bed for your loved one in a facility within your community. The kind of respite and length will depend on what you and your loved one would find most comfortable and helpful for your situation.

- Ask a friend or family member to visit your loved one more often while you go out.
- Your home care nurse may be able to advise or assist with organizing respite care. They can arrange short-term admission into a long-term care or hospice bed or for paid help in your home. This will depend on what is available in your community.

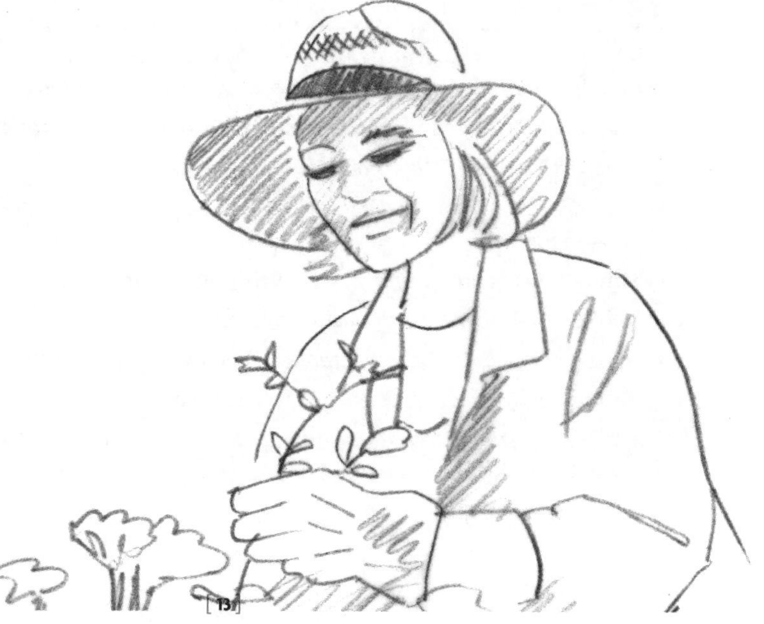

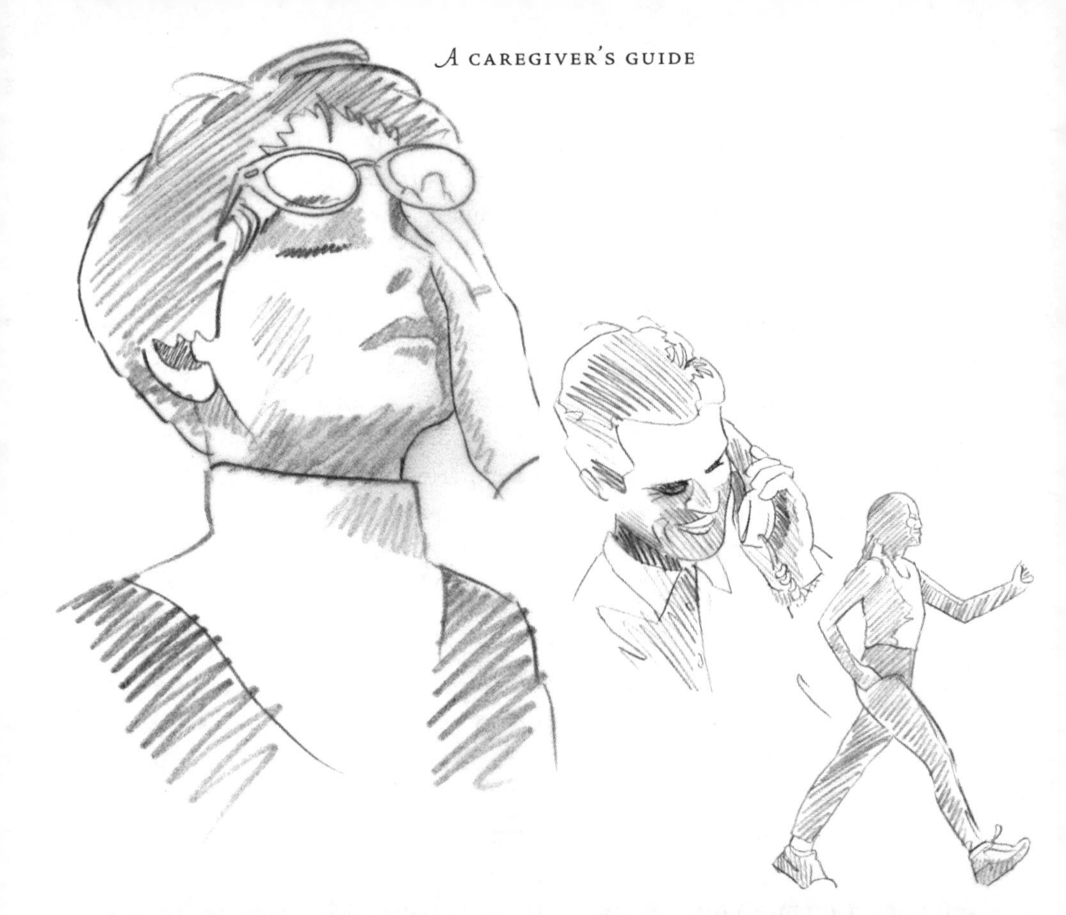

## IMPORTANT POINTS

**CAREGIVER "BURNOUT"**

*The word "burnout" describes the exhaustion of physical or emotional strength. It is a good description of the way you may feel sometimes.*
*Seek help if you find that any of the following are happening:*

- *The urge to run and hide from responsibility becomes strong.*
- *Your activity is scattered and frantic.*
- *There is a major change in your sleeping patterns such as sleeping less than three hours.*
- *Eating habits change and you suddenly gain or lose more than 10 pounds,*
- *You are often irritable or easily angered.*
- *Important details are forgotten or you cannot concentrate.*
- *You use extra alcohol, drugs or tobacco to cope.*

*Consider that some kind of respite may be what you need to keep going.*

Home help may be available to:

- come in at night to keep the person company while you sleep.
- give food or drinks to the person.
- help the person to move about in bed.
- just stay close to allow you to take time for yourself.

Take physical respite breaks by:

- going for a walk.
- working in your garden.
- sitting in your backyard.
- going for lunch with a friend.
- going to a movie.
- finding a restful place and being in the quiet.

Take mental respite breaks by:

- meditating.
- reading a book.
- listening to music
- watching television.
- doing handicrafts.
- talking to a friend.

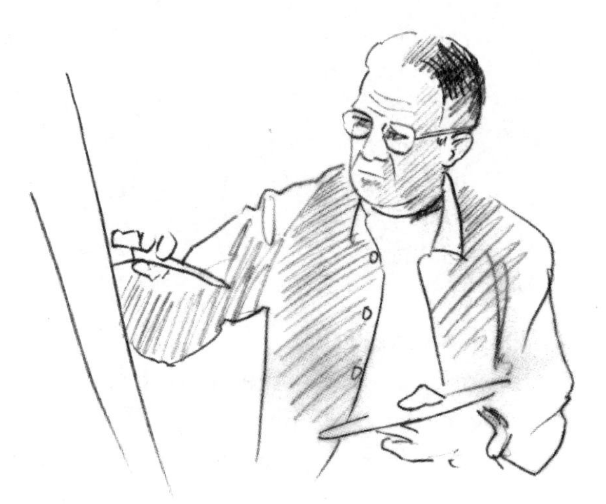

Nourish your spirit by:

- spending time in reflection.
- going to spiritual ceremonies, activities or services.
- talking to spiritual advisors.
- engaging in any spiritual activity that comforts you.

# SUPPORT NETWORKS

■

Caring for a person with a progressive life-threatening illness is not easy and requires people with different skills who can support you. These people could consist of both your formal health care team and/or informal group of family and friends. You and your loved one are always the central core in both support teams.

## IMPORTANT POINTS

- *Support networks may be there to help you and your loved one, but you may need to be specific about what you need at the time.*
- *Remember to reach out to find out what help is there for you. You do not need to try to do everything yourself.*
- *Make lists of questions and concerns about the person's care as they occur. Have them in front of you when you talk with friends and the health care team.*
- *Having helpers in the home always takes some adjustment. All of the family must adapt, even to visits from members of the healthcare team such as nurses or personal care workers. Let people know if you are struggling with it.*

### INFORMAL SUPPORT

To work out who would be considered your informal support group, first find out who may be willing or has offered to help. Sometimes help can come from unexpected sources outside of family and friends, such as co-workers or volunteers. You also need to be prepared that some family and friends will not want or are unable to be involved.

- Make a list of your daily routine, what needs to be done, who could help with different tasks, and post it in a clearly visible place. Remember those who want to support you often do not know your routine. They may hesitate to ask yet would be willing to do tasks such as making meals, changing the cat litter or doing laundry if they knew those were needed. Review and update your list on a regular basis.
- Ask directly for help with:
  - practical tasks such as shopping, meal preparation, housework, screening calls and providing information.
  - outdoor tasks such as mowing the lawn or shoveling the walkway.
  - picking up prescriptions or driving you to an appointment.

Find out when people are available to help.

- Some people to ask for help are:
  - family, friends, neighbours, or co-workers.
  - members from your social organizations or community.
  - minister, priest or other religious or spiritual advisers.
  - community agencies or volunteers who can visit to sit, chat, read aloud, play cards, or provide transportation.

### FORMAL SUPPORT

Your formal support network is more structured than the informal one. It may include:

- a family doctor who may perform home visits (always ask).
- a home care nurse.
- other members of the home care team such as occupational therapists, physiotherapists, social workers, respiratory therapists and volunteers.
- personal care workers or home support aides who provide care and can give you a break.
- pharmacists who can give you information on your medications and may be able to arrange for delivery to your home.
- a dietician who can advise on what foods or fluids are appropriate at different stages of the illness.
- community agencies that offer useful services such as paid respite support or volunteers. These services may include preparing meals, house cleaning, grocery shopping, shoveling walkways or mowing the lawn.

### PLEASE NOTE

Your family doctor can contact home care agencies or you may do so yourself. Someone will then visit your home to assess your needs. Home care programs provide different services in different locations. All home care programs have nurses but some may not include all of the services and professionals listed above.

Additional services offered may also include:

- emotional and bereavement support for you, your loved one and your family.
- visiting consult programs to help with pain and other symptoms.
- personal care such as bathing, feeding or moving the person.
- respite care.
- referrals to other community agencies.

# COMMUNICATION WITH OTHERS

## COMMUNICATING WITH YOUR LOVED ONE

Communication involves talking and most importantly listening. Communication is also the "gift of presence" which means simply being with a person and paying attention, without any expectations or need for conversation. Sometimes it may include sharing personal contact (with permission). Remember that gentle touching, holding, hugging and caressing are ways to express love, acceptance and caring connections that may be important for both of you.

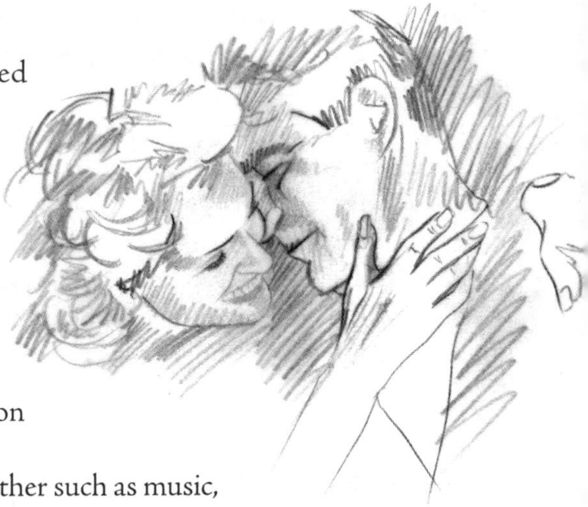

### Ideas to help you communicate

- Be an active and interested listener.
- Gently squeeze a hand or offer an embrace.
- Sit in silence. This can be as supportive as any conversation and requires less energy.
- Share and enjoy humor and happy memories.
- Do not let illness put a ban on smiles and laughter.
- Enjoy meaningful things together such as music, art, sports, movies, or audiobooks.
- Help your loved one stay in contact with friends and outside activities by assisting with phone calls, visits, and emails.
- Speak to each other about feelings, fears and concerns.
- Be aware that your loved one may be expressing anger and taking it out on you. If this happens often or you find it difficult to cope when it happens, it may be best to seek outside help.
- If your loved one is alert but cannot speak, your healthcare team may be able to assist you with obtaining a communication board.
- Consider reading books that may help you as you talk to your loved one, such as R. Buckman's *I Don't Know What To Say*.

## Guidelines for conversation/communication

- Think about how you and your loved one communicated before the illness, what worked and what may need help.
- Pay attention to what is being said, the tone of voice and body language, as well as the words themselves.
- Try different openings for conversation. You could start with an observation like, "You seem relaxed (tense) today." Asking if there is anything the person wants to talk about is another good way to start a conversation. Give broad openings so the conversation and topic can go many directions. For example: "Tell me more about . . ." or "What does it mean to you to . . .?"
- Be attentive and try not to let your mind wander to your own thoughts and reactions. Good listening takes concentration.
- Test your understanding by repeating back what you have just heard. This helps to keep things clear.
- Respect what the person chooses to talk about rather than taking the lead yourself.
- Encourage but don't push.
- Accept what the person is saying, however different it may be from what you think.
- Talk about what is important to you using "I" statements. An example would be, "I want to help and I need you to tell me how."
- Be honest while not being hurtful with your comments and observations.
- Encourage yet do not push your loved one to share thoughts and feelings.
- Be willing to say you do not know the answers to a particular question.
- Be aware that it is not uncommon for a loved one to return to the use of their mother tongue as death comes nears. If you do not speak the language, try to find someone who does.
- Listen carefully for meaningful questions and do your best to respond or call on someone who can.

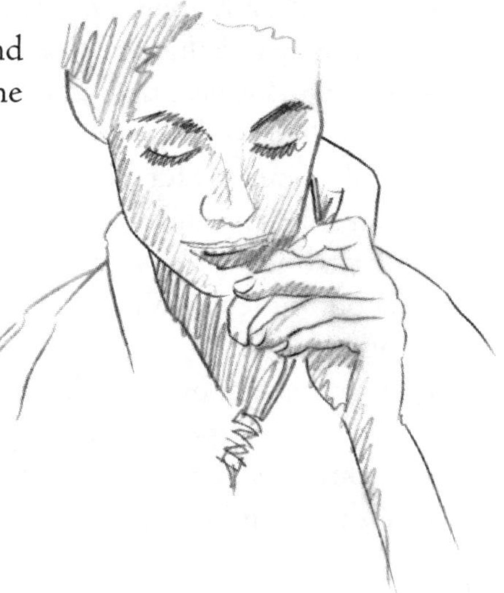

### Things to avoid

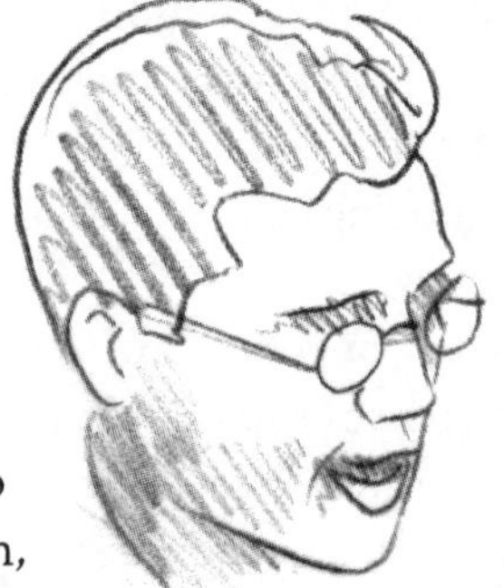

- Do not make promises you cannot keep or offer empty reassurances.
- Do not make judgments about what the person says, does or feels. Everyone has a right to their feelings and opinion, and that right should be respected.
- Do not avoid uncomfortable issues by changing the subject or introducing an unrelated topic. Express your discomfort and suggest that someone other than you may be better able to help.

## COMMUNICATING WITH OTHER FAMILY MEMBERS

When you care for someone with a progressive life threatening illness, you may need family support and communication from those members living close to you and also those at a distance. Let your family know how you want to communicate with them so that everyone can respond in ways that are helpful, understanding and comforting.

Some suggestions for family communication:

- Find ways to keep in touch with other family members by email and phone.
- Consider ways to record special family moments, events and gatherings.
- Talk to family about how you are doing and encourage them to do the same. You may be reluctant to express concerns for fear of hurting each other's feelings. Respect that certain family members may not wish to talk about all feelings and thoughts.
- Talk about the future and make important decisions while your loved one can still be included.
- Let family know what you need and when you need it. For instance, talk about the length and frequency of their visits, and how they can help you in other ways.
- Reminisce about your lives together, the best and worst moments, family strengths, important times and events.
- Acknowledge and deal with changes in family roles and responsibilities.
- Ask for family help to learn new and unfamiliar tasks.

## COMMUNICATING WITH CHILDREN

Children understand illness, death and dying in different ways at different age levels. You may communicate better with your children by using reading materials or asking a professional to give you guidance on children's understanding on illness and death at various ages. It is important to give all children opportunities to understand what is happening, ask questions and express their feelings.

- Learn what the children already understand and know.
- Tell the truth and do not try to "spare" your children from knowing that a loved one is dying. Children may not understand all that is going on in the home. However, they will sense and feel tension, stress, anxiety, sadness and secrets in the adults around them.
- Children can be surprisingly strong and adaptable to difficult situations, provided they are permitted to ask questions, express their feelings and have an avenue of open communication with their family. Whispered conversations behind closed doors can make them imagine situations that are worse than reality.
- Include children in activities with their loved one, but never force their involvement. Just make suggestions and then let them decide.
- Consider short visits, especially for younger children.
- Ensure that the child's school is aware that a loved one is gravely ill or dying.
- Reserve separate time for the children to read or play, go on outings or just be together.
- Be consistent and maintain routines.
- Consider using some of the excellent books that are available to help you discuss illness, dying, death, grief and loss with your children. (see Books to Help Grieving Children, page 138).

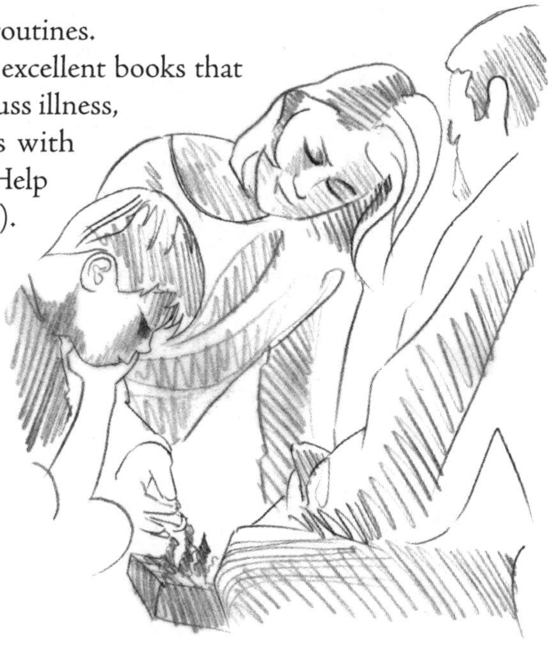

## COMMUNICATING WITH THE HEALTH CARE TEAM

It is good to have regular and open communication with your loved one's doctor, nurse and other health care providers. Remember that final decisions about care rest primarily in the hands of the person who is ill, unless the ability to make decisions is gone. It is wise to complete an advance care plan. Appoint someone else, such as a substitute health decision maker, to speak for loved ones if they cannot speak for themselves. Use the advice you get from the health care team as a starting point for discussion.

**What you need to consider:**

- As you and your loved one think of questions, write them down for your health care team member(s). When it is time to ask the questions, either record the answers yourself or have someone do it for you so you can review them later.
- Try to deal with several concerns in one meeting with the health care provider. Think about what you need to know and who might be the best person to provide assistance.
- Make sure you understand the advice and answers you are given. Ask questions to clarify before the visit or phone call ends.
- Tell your health care team immediately about any new pains or symptoms of your loved one, so they can be dealt with quickly.
- Tell the doctor or nurse about any medical or complementary therapies your loved one may be using. This is extremely important as there may be serious side effects when used with other medications or treatments.
- Once a decision on a treatment plan and goals of care with interventions are mutually agreed upon, follow the advice given. Remember that these decisions and choices can be reviewed at any time.
- Remember that, depending on your local community health care team resources, various members of your health care team may also be there to help with your emotional and spiritual needs.

### COMMUNICATING WITH VISITORS

When friends and family know that their loved one has a progressive illness they may want to connect more often and spend extra time with that person. Here are some basic guidelines to help:

- Talk with your loved one about visitors ahead of time. Discuss who they may wish to see, how often and for how long. Use this as your initial guide to communicate with visitors, while letting them know that your loved one's desires for company may change over time as their condition changes.
- Give a time limit for the visit.
- Encourage visitors to phone first and check if it is a good time to come to visit.
- Suggest that visitors just sit quietly or talk in a way that does not require answers, especially if talking causes breathlessness or tires your loved one.
- Discourage anyone who may be sick (especially with a cold or flu) from visiting. This includes if they have recently been in contact with someone who is sick.
- Put a sign on your entrance door or a message on your phone letting people know when you or your loved one is not able to receive visitors.
- Consider having a guest book so you can keep track and remember all who visited.

Find out ahead of time if there is a topic that visitors may want to explore and whether or not your loved one wishes to discuss it. Let visitors know the response, and give an update on your loved one's condition and what to expect before the visit.

## SPIRITUAL NEEDS

■

For some people, spirituality is how they see themselves in relation to others, the earth and the universe. For others, a spiritual power is at the heart of these relationships. That spiritual power may vary according to cultural belief systems. Those who embrace this type of spirituality often do so within an organized religion. Even within a specific religion people may have differing ways of relating to their spiritual power. For these reasons, the spiritual needs of a person with a progressive life threatening illness may be obvious at times and not so obvious at others.

A common spiritual desire is the search for the meaning and purpose of living and dying, hoping for miracles or searching for immortality. Some people understand or seek meaning for what is happening within the context of their spiritual or religious belief, while others look elsewhere.

You may feel you know your loved one's beliefs. Still, you need to reach out and explore that with your loved one, especially at this time of facing and coming to terms with a progressive illness.

**What you need to understand:**

- Your loved one may have lost contact with their faith community or spiritual power and want to return or reconnect. They may no longer find comfort in previously held beliefs or spiritual relationships.
- People sometimes express guilt, remorse and a desire for forgiveness in a search for inner peace.
- In trying to make sense of what is happening people may ask "Why?" internally or externally, either of their spiritual power or the universe at large.

**How you can offer spiritual comfort:**

- Consider your comfort level with your own as well as your loved one's spirituality.
- Be sure to respect and support your loved one's spiritual needs at this time.
- Help a loved one who wishes to pray but can't remember how, even if prayer does not come easily. Knowing that prayers can be offered in that person's name by others may be a consolation.
- With your loved one's permission, share news of the illness with their spiritual community and ask if they can be available as spiritual companions if called upon.
- Do not feel obligated to offer your own answers to any searching questions the person asks of a spiritual power. It is most important to be there as a caring listener and understanding supporter.

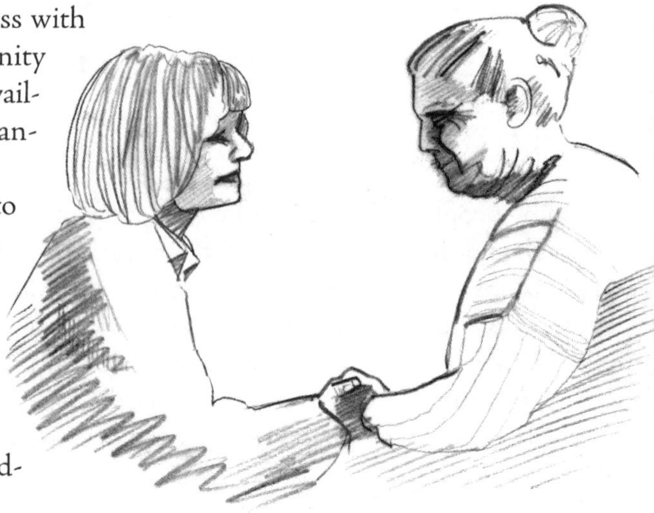

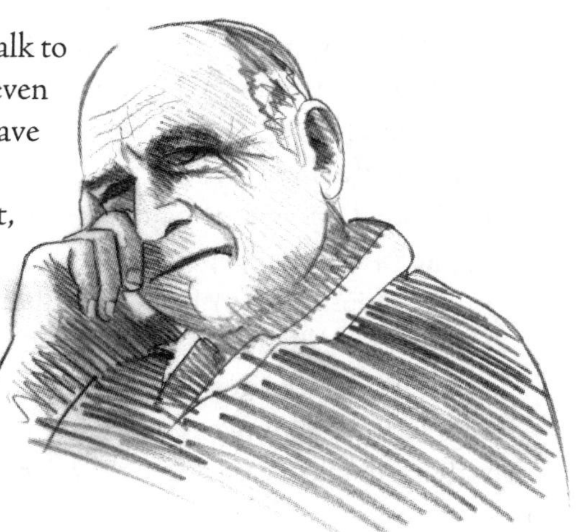

- Ask the person if it would help to talk to someone about spiritual matters, even if this type of contact may not have been important before now.
- If your loved one is feeling doubt, guilt, anger, disbelief, uncertainty, a sense of resignation, acceptance, healing or peace, reassure that these and other mixed emotions can be normal feelings at this time.
- Be prepared to listen, support and accept if and when the person expresses a need to do some life review, talk about death, and prepare to say goodbyes.
- Reach out for your own spiritual resources to help you if and when you feel the need.

Although they may not say it out loud, those who are ill may wonder if their life has been meaningful to those they love and whether they will be remembered. Keep in mind that there may be special spiritual reflection times and opportunities where you can share the importance of what your loved one's life has meant to you and the many memories that you will continue to carry on.

## ADAPTING YOUR HOME

■

When caring for someone at home, you need to consider the location in the home where most of the care will be provided. The home care nurse or occupational therapist can make recommendations about adapting your home based on some of the following questions:

- Will the person spend most of their time in bed?
- Will they prefer to stay in their bedroom or closer to family activities?
- Is it necessary to have a bathroom close by?
- Can the person walk far or climb stairs?

### How you can offer comfort and care

With a few changes to household arrangements, you may be able to adapt your home without too much trouble.

- Avoid having rugs on the floor, as they slip easily and could cause a fall.
- Create an area, near a window if possible, surrounded by favorite mementoes, music and pets.
- Keep helpful items within reach such as:
    - A small table at the height of the bed for tissues, medication, snacks, radio, and notepaper.
    - A comfortable armchair nearby that is high enough to get in and out of easily.
    - A small bell, baby monitor or buzzer to call for help.
    - Seating for visitors.

Ask the home care nurse or occupational therapist about home aids and equipment that can make care at home easier. Many of these may be available to rent in your area.

Some examples of home aids and equipment include:

- a hospital bed.
- bed rails (full or half length).
- overbed table.
- alternating pressure mattress.
- bedpan/slipper pan/urinal.
- commode.
- hair washing tray.
- raised toilet seat/ toilet with arm rest.
- supportive mattress or cushion.
- walker.
- wheelchair.
- cane.
- crutches.
- foam cushion.
- back rest.
- bolster/wedge.
- bath rail.
- bath board.
- bath lift.
- bath chair.
- floor to ceiling pole.
- transfer belt or rented mechanical or battery-powered lifts.

CHAPTER

# 2

# GIVING PHYSICAL CARE

# INFECTION CONTROL (UNIVERSAL PRECAUTIONS)

■

Universal precautions protect you and the person you are caring for from infection. Infection control is important, as anyone may carry any number of bacteria (germs). Precautions apply to everyone. You may need equipment like as gloves, aprons and masks, which can be purchased from your pharmacist or a business that sells health supplies. Costs related to these products may be covered by some programs. Your home care nurse can provide advice and precautions on how to use gloves, wash surfaces or use specialized puncture-proof containers to dispose of sharp objects. Be sure to wash soiled linens in hot water separate from other laundry, and use bleach and a dryer on high if necessary.

## HANDWASHING

Washing your hands is the most effective way to prevent the spread of infections. Wash them with warm soapy water before and after every contact with the person for whom you are caring. Keep nails and cuticles trimmed so your hands are easy to keep clean. Prevent dryness and chapping with hand lotion. You can also use alcohol-based waterless antiseptic if hands are not visibly soiled, alternating wash hands with soap and water.

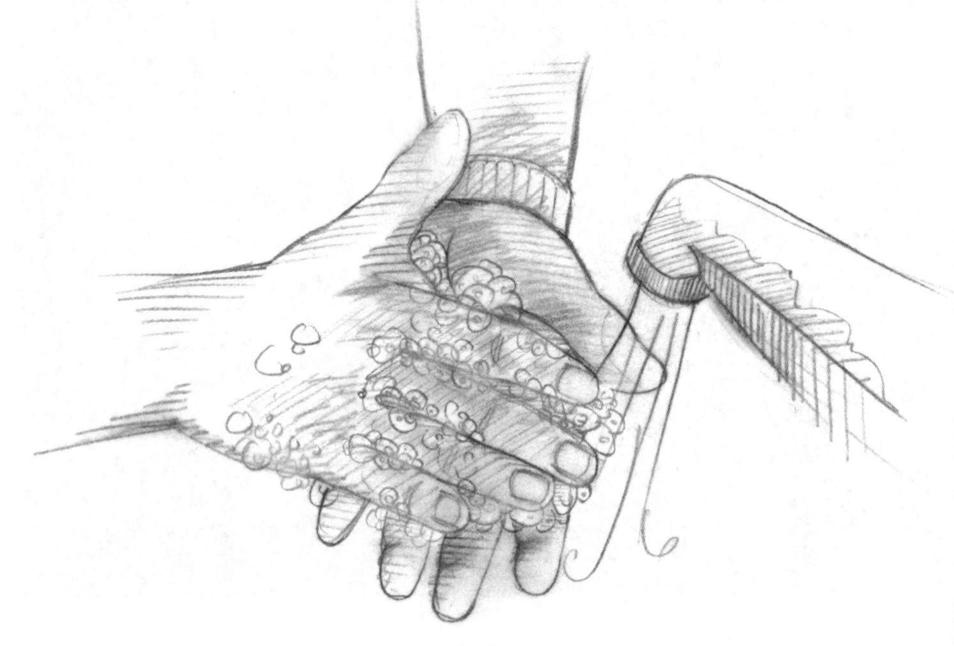

### GARBAGE DISPOSAL

All dirty dressings or used disposable products with blood or body fluids on them must be placed inside two plastic bags for disposal. This will contain all of the bacteria to avoid infection.

### GLOVES

Disposable latex or vinyl gloves should be worn to handle objects that have blood or body fluids on them. Disposable gloves should never be reused or left out, and should be put in two plastic bags in the garbage.

### APRONS

Wear a disposable plastic apron if your clothes are likely to be soiled while you give care. Place the apron in the two plastic bags in the garbage when you take it off.

### MASKS

Wear a mask if you have a cold. If the person you are caring for is coughing a lot, you may also choose to wear a mask. Ask your home care nurse how to use the mask properly.

### NEEDLES AND SYRINGES

Place used needles and syringes in a hard plastic or metal container with a lid. Place the lid on the container when it is full and tape it shut so the needles will not fall out and stick anyone. The procedure for disposal varies across each province, so ask your home care nurse how it is done in your community. Clearly label the container with an alert as to what it contains.

### FOOD PREPARATION

Raw foods are prime carriers of germs. Meats and eggs should be cooked thoroughly. Always wash fruits and vegetables before you cook or eat them. Wash dishes, glassware and cooking utensils in hot, soapy water. If you use a cutting board to prepare raw meat, always wash and sanitize the board in hot water and vinegar before you use it again. Keep surfaces clean and dry.

### PETS

Since animals can carry disease, it is important to make sure that family pets are healthy and up to date for check-ups or shots. Make sure you wash your hands thoroughly after you clean the cat's litter box or the bird's cage.

# BATHING

■

Bathing is an important part of personal care and offers both physical and emotional comfort.

### How you can offer care

Someone who is strong enough to move about can be helped to wash in a shower, bathtub, or at the sink.

- Put a bath chair on a non-slip mat in the tub or shower if getting in and out or standing for a long time is difficult. A chair at the sink can also be used.
- Ask your home care nurse or occupational therapist for advice as to how to make the bathroom safer and easier to use. Equipment such as bars, non-slip surfaces and bath lifts (if available) may be helpful.
- Before helping the person into the bathroom, gather all the things you will need such as:
  - clean clothes or pajamas.
  - soap, shaving supplies and shampoo.
  - face cloth.
  - towel.
  - lotion.
- Test the water temperature of the bath or shower.
- Help the person to get into the bath or shower.
- Allow the person to wash as much as possible. You may need to help with the back, legs, feet and genital area.
- Offer assistance out of the bath or shower and help to dry. A bath towel put in the dryer for a few minutes before it is needed can provide added warmth.
- Help the person into clean clothes.

## BED BATH

Someone who must stay in bed will benefit from a bed bath every day. As well as providing cleanliness, it refreshes your loved one and gives you the chance to connect, talk and listen.

### How you can offer care

Although a bed bath can be given at any time, people who are ill often have more energy for a bath in the morning. Ask the person what time would be best. Talk as you help with the bathing, advising on what you are going to do next like washing left foot or right arm. Remember to separate hair washing time from bathing time as it may be tiring to do it all together.

- Provide privacy.
- Gather the things you will need:
  - large bowl with warm water.
  - soap.
  - wash cloth and towels.
  - light bed cover.
  - lotion.
- If possible, raise the level of the bed to lessen the strain on your back.
- Cover the person with a light sheet or blanket for warmth. Only uncover and wash one part of the body at a time.
- Put dry towels under the body part being washed to keep the person and bed linen dry.
- Use a gentle soap or bath oil on the skin, then rinse and dry.
- Start at the face and work down towards the feet.
- Wash the chest, legs, arms and sides first, and then help the person to lie on one side while you wash the back.
- Apply lotion if desired after drying an area.
- Change wash clothes and water, then wash the genital and anal areas last. It is important that these areas be cleaned well at least daily, as bacteria tend to collect there. Wash between the person's legs from the front toward the back. If cloth becomes soiled use another clean cloth and rinse well.
- Apply a water-repellent cream (e.g. Penaten Cream™, Zincofax™, A&D Cream™) to the genital area if incontinence is a problem.
- Change the water as often as necessary to keep it clean and hot. Keep the washbasin clean and dry between bed baths to reduce the risk of infection.

- Apply lotion to all pressure areas. While you are using the lotion, the person may appreciate a complete back rub. (see Attention to Skin Pressure Areas, page 36).
- Change sheet during and after the bed bath is finished. (see Making a Bed with Someone in it, page 41).
- If a complete bed bath is too tiring, wash the person's face, hands, back, underarms and genitals daily.
- Remember shaving, make-up and brushing and styling hair are important parts of care and will help the person feel more comfortable. Often a rest before and after these activities will help prevent the person from becoming over-tired.
- Ensure that items like reading glasses and hearing aids are returned within reach of the person at the end of the bed bath.
- The bed linens should be changed at the same time as the bed bath.

## IMPORTANT POINTS

- *If movement causes pain, give pain medication about 30 minutes before the bath.*
- *Avoid powder as it tends to cake in body creases.*
- *Home support workers may be available for personal care help.*

# MOUTH CARE

■

Cleaning a person's mouth is not difficult. By helping your loved one have a clean mouth, you will increase comfort, prevent mouth sores and make eating and drinking easier.

## How you can offer care

### Brushing teeth

- Help the person into a sitting position. If it is more comfortable, or if the person cannot sit, raise the head of the bed.
- Place a dry towel under the chin. Have a bowl handy – it can also be placed under the chin if tolerated.
- Give the person a sip of water to moisten the inside of the mouth.
- Use an ultra-soft toothbrush and soften the bristles in hot water.
- Do not use toothpaste as it can be harsh on fragile gum tissue. Moisten the brush in one of the rinsing solutions suggested later in this section under Rinsing.
- Brush the teeth using gentle strokes starting at the gum line and moving to the edge of the teeth.
- Brush the cheeks, gums and tongue gently.
- Do not put the toothbrush too near the back of the throat as this may cause gagging.
- Try to remove all food particles and crusted material.
- Have the person rinse with cool water and spit into the bowl or basin.
- If the person is unconscious, brush with caution. A soft toothbrush moistened in one of the rinsing solutions or a toothette (a swab with a sponge head - see warning alert under Important Points). Gently rub along the teeth, gums and tongue.

## DENTURE CARE

- If the person has dentures, remove these and clean them with a toothbrush.
- Do not use very hot water on dentures as they may warp.
- Do not soak dentures in bleach as this may damage them. Any commercially available product marketed for denture soaking may be used.
- If the gums are dry under dentures, a product such as Oral Balance™ may provide comfort.

- If dentures are loose or poor fitting, they may cause mouth sores. Have them refitted by a denturist or, if this is not possible, leave them out except when eating.

## LIP CARE

- Put a water-soluble lubricant such as K-Y Jelly™, Muco™ or Dermabase™ on the lips.
- Avoid using oil-based products such as Vaseline™, Chapstick™ and mineral oil. These may make open sores on the lips more inflamed.

## RINSING

- Rinsing the mouth is not a substitute for brushing.
- If the person is not able to get out of bed, aim to rinse the mouth at the same time you do skin care. For an unconscious person, wipe the mouth with a gauze dipped in a rinsing solution or with a toothette.
- Use a non-alcohol based rinsing solution. Suggestions include:
  - baking soda (1 teaspoon) and water (2 cups).
  - salt (½ teaspoon), baking soda (1 teaspoon) and water (4 cups).
  - club soda.
- Avoid over-the-counter mouthwashes that contain alcohol. The alcohol can make mouth tissue dry and increase the risk of infection.

## IMPORTANT POINTS

- *As many bacteria grow in the mouth, wash your hands well before and after you give mouth care.*
- *Although toothettes are a convenient way to clean a person's mouth, they can break apart while in the mouth. Use them with caution.*
- *Do not give mouth care to a person who is lying flat as this may cause choking. For someone unable to raise the head, help to turn to the side and wipe any moisture remaining in the mouth with a gauze, clean cloth or toothette.*
- *If the person bites down on the toothbrush or toothette, do not let go or try to yank it out. The jaw will eventually relax and you will be able to remove it.*
- *Check in the person's mouth every day for signs of sores or other problems* (see *Mouth Problems*, page 82).
- *Do not put your fingers in the mouth of a person who is confused or sleepy. You run the risk of being bitten.*
- *Mouth care should be done at least twice a day.*

# POSITIONING SOMEONE IN BED

■

If someone is completely bedridden, too weak to move, paralysed or unconscious, changing the position in bed will become one of your most important tasks. Long periods without moving can lead to pressure sores, which is a serious problem. Also, changing position helps keep the lungs free of mucus longer and can help ease pain.

## How you can offer care

Often when a person finds a comfortable position, it is a strong temptation to stay there without moving. You may need to insist when helping your loved one to shift in bed. Ensure you have the supplies you need, such as pillows, close at hand.

- Lower the head of the bed if this is possible.
- Loosen the bed covers and remove extra pillows.
- Move the person toward you on one side of the bed, so that after the turn the person will be in the centre of the bed. (See Figure 1.)
- Use a turning sheet (sometimes called a draw sheet, page 39) to help roll the person over (see Helping Someone Move Up in Bed, page 38).
- If you do not have a turning sheet:
  - Stand on the opposite side of the bed from where the person is lying.
  - Place the person's far arm across the chest towards you. (See Figure 2.)
  - Bend the far leg at the knee and bring the bent leg towards you. As you do this, the far shoulder will naturally start to move towards you. Place your hand behind the person's shoulder and roll the body toward yourself. Do not pull the person's arm while doing this. (See Figure 3.)
  - Place the person's knees and ankles together in a flexed position.
- Place a flat pad or pillow under the knees and lower legs.

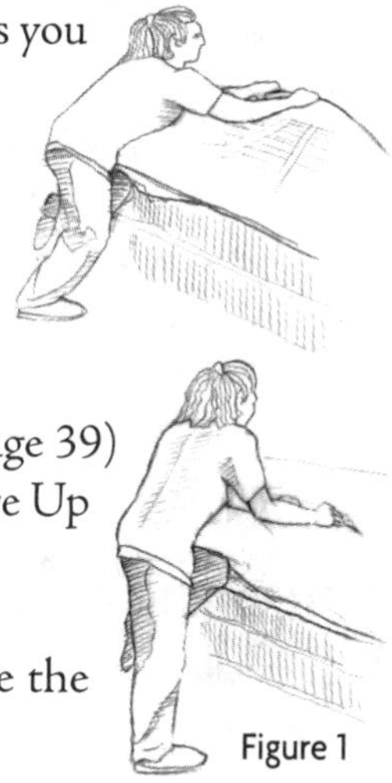

Figure 1

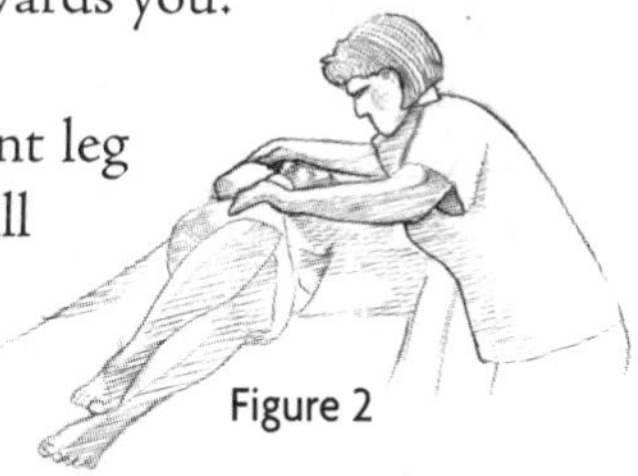

Figure 2

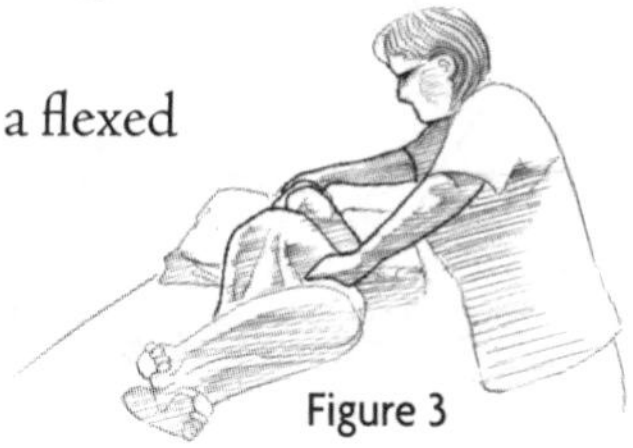

Figure 3

- Place a pillow lengthwise at the person's back and anchor it by pushing the edge underneath the back. Fold the outer side of the pillow under and tuck it in snugly against the person to give more support.
- Place a pillow lengthways under the person's thigh, bringing the leg forward so it does not rest on the lower leg. Position the leg comfortably.
- Place another pillow lengthways under the person's lower leg to prevent skin surfaces from rubbing together and to provide correct support. The pillow should extend well under the foot so the ankle and the foot do not drop and are kept level.
- Make sure the lower arm is in a comfortable position. The upper arm and hand may be more comfortable if placed on a pillow.
- When positioning someone on the back:
  - Place two pillows lengthways at an angle. They should extend under the person's shoulders.
  - Place one pillow across the top of the two lengthways pillows so it is under the head and reaching to the shoulders. (See Figure 4.)
  - A bar above the bed called a monkey or trapeze bar is a device that can help with moving in bed if the person has good upper body strength. Ask your home care nurse or occupational therapist if this would be helpful or available.

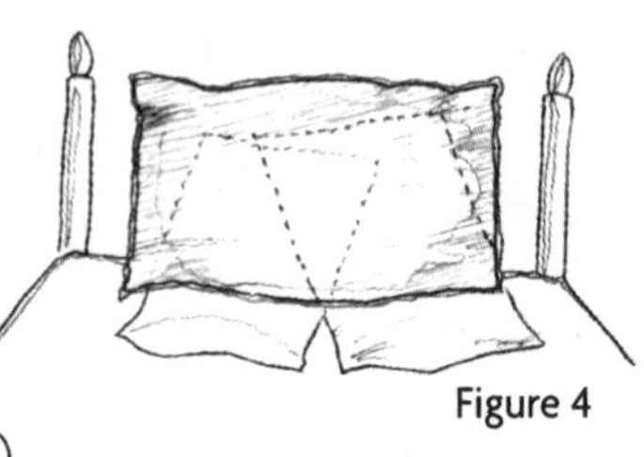
Figure 4

## ATTENTION TO SKIN PRESSURE AREAS

Skin breakdown or pressure sores can be a major source of discomfort for your loved one. Prevention of sores is a major part of physical care.

- Pressure sores usually happen over bony areas. (See Figure 5.)
- A regular back rub promotes blood supply to bony areas and can be relaxing as well.
- Encourage a person who can move unaided to change position in a bed or chair at least every two hours.

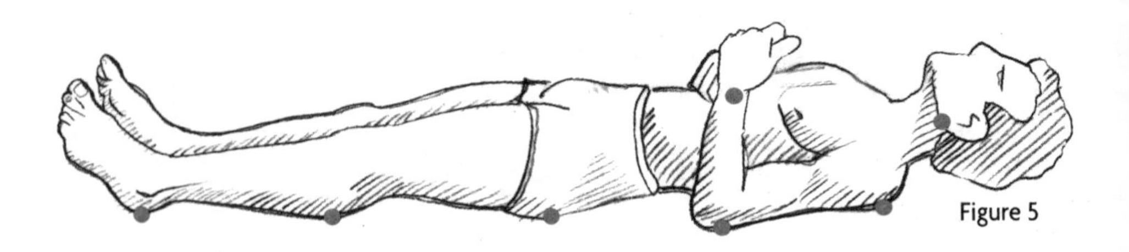
Figure 5

- Help a person who cannot move alone to turn every two hours during the daytime and every four hours at night. This routine may vary depending on the symptoms and stage of the illness. Seek guidance from the health care team.
- Ask your home care nurse about using a mattress or cushions that could help prevent pressure.
- Check the skin for any reddened areas as these may turn into pressure sores. (This can be done during the bed bath).
- Massage the back and pressure areas with lotion after each turn. Use soft pressure and move your hands in a circular motion.
- Do this several times, using plenty of lotion so that the movement is smooth.
- Protect reddened areas with pillows, and elbow and heel protectors. Ask your home care nurse about these and other protective devices such as special mattresses.
- Use pillows to support the person lying in a side position. The pillows can be gradually pulled away, so that after two hours the person rolls to the back.
- Keep the skin clean and dry.
- Keep bed sheets dry and free of wrinkles.

# HELPING SOMEONE MOVE UP IN BED

■

As a person gets weaker it may be necessary to provide help to move in bed.

## IMPORTANT POINTS

- *Give pain medication about 30 minutes before turning if movement causes pain.*
- *Do not rub any reddened areas that remain red after you have changed the person's position. Tell your home care nurse about these areas.*
- *When helping a person to move, do not drag. Dragging causes friction, which can cause skin to tear.*
- *Though the person may have discomfort when being turned, it is important to try to maintain a turning routine, depending on the stage of the illness.*

### How you can offer care

- Someone who is lying in bed for long periods may need help shifting to a different comfortable position.
- If the bed has wheels, make sure the bed brakes are on and lower the head of the bed.
- Raise the bed to about your waist level. If the bed cannot be raised, remember to use your knees (not your back) when lifting.
- If the bed has side rails, lower the side rail closest to you.
- Check that no tubes or urine bags will be pulled with the move.
- Remove extra pillows and place a pillow against the headboard.

## MOVING WITH ONE PERSON

- Face the direction of the move. Your feet should be wide apart, toes pointing in the direction of the move. You can also place one knee on the bed to get close to the person. (See Figure 6.)
- Bend the person's knees. Place one hand under the person's back and other hand under the thighs.
- Enlist the help of the person.

Figure 6

- Count to three and work together - the person (with knees bent) pushes upwards as you lift towards the head of the bed.
- Do not pull the arms while you are helping with this positioning.

## MOVING WITH A TURNING SHEET

- Fold an extra sheet in half twice to use as a turning sheet or draw sheet. Place the sheet under the person so it goes from mid-thigh to shoulder.
- Bend the person's knees.
- Stand beside the bed near the person's head, facing the feet.
- Grasp the turning sheet with one hand on each side of the person's shoulders.
- Enlist the help of the person.
- Count to three and work together - the person (with knees bent) pushes upwards as you lift toward the head of the bed.

## MOVING WITH TWO PEOPLE

- Both people face the direction of the move on opposite sides of the bed. (See Figure 7.)
- Bend the person's knees.
- Both people place their hands under the person's shoulders and waist.
- Count to three and work together - the person in bed pushes upwards (bending the knees and using the heels) while the other two lift toward the head of the bed.
- If a turning or draw sheet is being used, grasp the sheet on each side close to the person's shoulders and hips.
- On the count of three, the person (with knees bent) pushes upwards and the other two lift toward the head of the bed. (See Figure 8.)

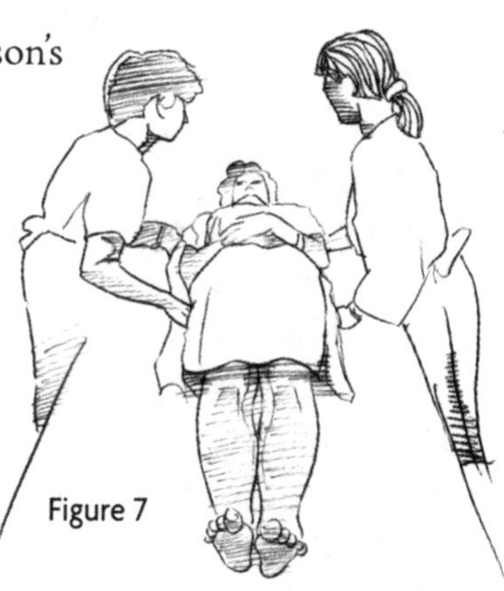

Figure 7

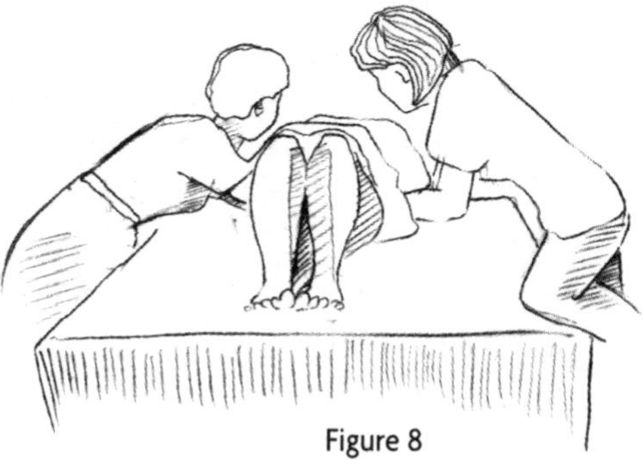

Figure 8

# MAKING A BED

■

For someone who is ill, the bed is often a place of refuge and comfort. If your loved one is confined to bed, the bedroom is the centre of activity and should be kept clean, tidy and restful.

## How you can offer comfort and care

It is important that the bed and surrounding area be kept clean to protect your loved one from problems such as bedsores or infections. Change the sheets at least once a week and whenever they are soiled.

- Start by asking the person if this is a good time for you to change the bed. Wait for another time if tiredness or symptoms seem to be a problem.
- Ask the person if it is possible to sit in a chair for a few moments while you change the bed (see if this is included in *Notes for you and your nurse*, page 180).
- Give a pain medication if needed, then wait about 30 minutes before you start.
- Collect the clean bedding and take it to the bedside. Place it on a nearby chair.
- Have a laundry basket or bags close by so you can put soiled bedding directly into them.
- Raise the bed to your waist level if this is possible. Lower the head of the bed so the bed is level.
- Remove the soiled bedding and place it in the laundry basket. Check that the mattress is dry and clean.
- Place a moisture-absorbing mattress sheeting or pad across the middle or full section of the mattress to protect it from moisture, especially if the person has diarrhea or is incontinent. Your home care nurse or local pharmacy may be able to tell you about other products available in your community.
- Be sure the sheets are flat and free of wrinkles to help prevent skin breakdown.
- Consider placing a turning or draw sheet over the bottom sheet. This can assist with lifting and turning while protecting the bottom sheet from becoming soiled, saving you from changing the entire bed. A flannel sheet or light blanket folded in half can serve as a turning or draw sheet.
- Place the clean top sheet and blankets on the bed. When tucking in the top layers, leave a little slack at the foot of the bed so the covers do not push down on the person's feet. If you are using a foot cradle, put it in place before you add the top layers.

- Replace the pillowcases daily or when soiled, tucking loose ends inside.
- If using incontinence pads, place a fresh one on the bottom sheet where the person's bottom will lie.
- Lower hospital bed to average bed height when you are finished.
- Help the person back to bed.
- Remove garbage such as used tissues.

## MAKING A BED WITH SOMEONE IN IT

When a person cannot get out of bed it is easier to have two people to help change it.

- Collect fresh bedding, laundry basket and bags. If using a hospital bed, raise the bed to waist level and lower the head so the bed is level with the person.
- Remove the top sheets, blankets and all pillows except the one that remains under the person's head. Cover the person with a sheet for warmth and privacy.
- Loosen the top and bottom sheets all around the bed.
- Help the person to turn onto one side while giving support at the waist and shoulders. Make sure the person's head is resting on a pillow and the limbs are supported (see Positioning Someone in Bed, page 35).
- If two of you are making the bed, one holds the person while the other rolls each layer of the bottom linens toward the centre of the bed, close to the person's back. If the person has been incontinent, take this chance to do a wash, then cover the soiled linens with a towel.
- If you are on your own, place a non-slip chair on the opposite side of the bed from you for the person to safely hold. If you have a hospital bed, raise the side rail and have the person hold on to that.
- Place the clean bottom sheet, rolled up lengthwise against the rolled-up dirty linens. Smooth out the flat half of the clean sheet and tuck it in. Repeat this process with each bottom layer of bedding you are using (mattress or foam, moisture-absorbing sheeting, bottom sheet, draw sheet, turning sheet, incontinence pads). This will form a small hump. (see Figure 9, page 42).

- Move the pillow to the other side of the bed. Help the person move and turn over the rolls of bedding to the other side. Make sure to warn about the hump.
- If there are two of you, the other person now pulls through all the dirty linens and places them in a used linen basket or bag.
- If changing the bed linens at the same time as the bed bath, finish washing the person, then change the pajamas prior to pulling all layers of the clean linens through. Pull tightly to make the bottom straight and wrinkle free, then tuck in the clean sheets (see Figure 9, page 42).
- Help the person into a comfortable position. Replace the pillowcases and finish making the bed with a top sheet, cover and blankets if needed.
- Empty and return the laundry basket to their regular places. Remember to wash your hands.

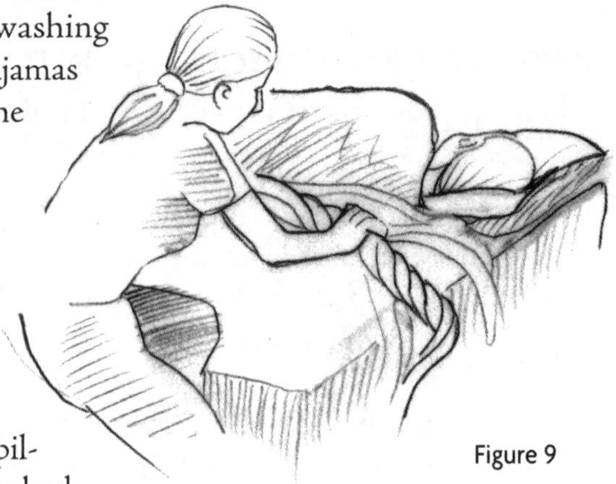

Figure 9

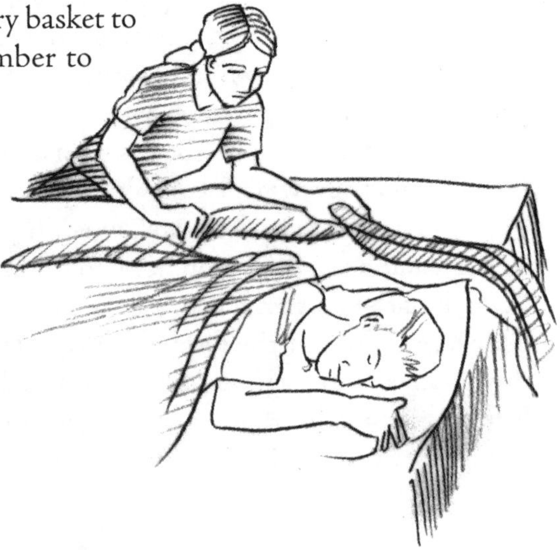

# HELPING WITH MOVING ABOUT

■

## BODY MECHANICS (USING YOUR BODY CORRECTLY)

Body mechanics refers to the way you use your body during movement. It is especially important when you are doing something that can strain your joints. Paying attention to body mechanics during lifting or bending will help to prevent injury. A member of your health care team can show you how to do the movements safely on your own using equipment or aids such as transfer boards, transfer belts poles, arm rests and side rails, if available.

### What you need to know

The most important aspect of your own body mechanics is knowledge of your body's abilities. Pay attention to your own limitations. There are three terms you need to understand.

1. Your centre of gravity is located at the middle of your body, about your hips.
2. Your line of balance is an imaginary line, from head to foot, that divides your body into two equal parts.
3. The base of support is the space between your feet that bears the weight of your body. (See Figure 10.)

- When moving or lifting anything heavy, reduce the strain on your back by keeping your line of balance close to your centre of gravity. Bend your knees instead of your back to keep from leaning forward or backward.
- Open the distance between your feet to broaden your base of support. This distributes the extra weight you are bearing or lifting and reduces strain on your back muscles.
- Get close to the object or person you are moving. Make sure your centres of gravity are as close as possible.
- Use your arm and leg muscles, not your back, to do the work. When using your arms, keep the load close to your body. Your greatest lift power comes with pushing rather than pulling.
- Look at where you are and where you want to go. Think through the movement before you proceed.

Figure 10

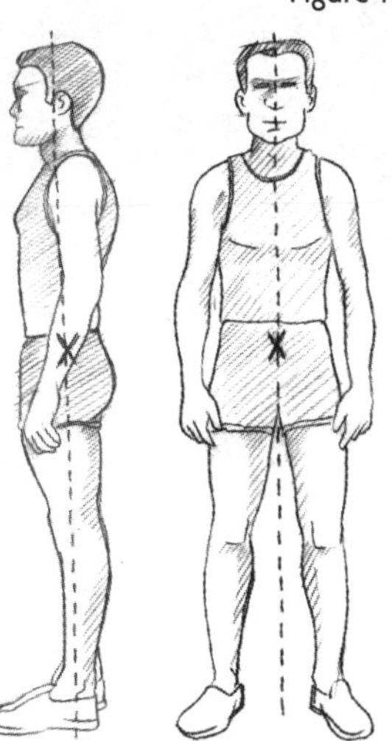

## LIFTING

When lifting a person, a few basic techniques done correctly can help prevent injury to everyone involved.

- Make sure obstacles or barriers are moved out of the way.
- Talk through the lift step by step so everyone involved understands the direction and purpose of the movement.
- Count to three before the movement begins, so everyone moves at the same time.
- Take a deep breath before you start and breathe regularly while lifting.
- Turn with your feet, pivot or step to avoid twisting your body.
- Always do the least amount of work to achieve your move. Have the person in bed help you as much as possible. Ask your home care nurse for advice about the availability of a transfer belt or other transfer aids for use.

### IMPORTANT POINTS

- *Do not attempt a lift that you think you cannot do alone. Two people are almost always better than one.*
- *If your back is weak or hurt do not attempt to lift or move someone.*
- *If you injure yourself, see your doctor right away.*
- *If the person begins to fall, do not resist the fall. Go with it gently and protect both of you from injury. Make sure to protect the person's head from hitting the floor.*
- *Once you reach the floor, take a few seconds to calm down and check that both of you are all right. Call for help if needed.*
- *To help up from a fall, move the person to a chair first and then from the chair to the bed. Start with the person kneeling, then holding onto a chair and rising from there.*

# MOVING SOMEONE FROM BED TO CHAIR

Getting out of bed when able can help lift the spirit as well as prevent bedsores.

## How you can offer care

- Take your time. A person who has been lying in bed for any length of time may feel dizzy when first sitting up.
- Make sure the dizziness has passed before making the move.
- Have all your equipment ready for the move. Put bed brakes on and lower the bed to chair height if that is possible.
- If the person is weaker on one side, place the chair on the stronger side. Otherwise place the chair at the head of the bed, facing the foot. If you are using a wheelchair, make sure the brakes are on. When possible, remove the armrest and foot pedal closest to the bed. (See Figure 11.)
- Make sure you and the person are both wearing non-slip footwear.
- Raise the head of the bed as high as it will go.
- Sit the person up in bed and move the legs over the side of the bed. Next, help the person slide forward to the edge of the bed. If you have a bed that can be lowered, the feet should touch the floor or if not, a safe nonslip footstool. (See Figure 12.)
- Keeping your back straight, bend your knees and lean towards the person.
- Put the person's arms around your back, not around your neck. If someone is too weak to grasp, place the arms over your shoulder with the head resting on your shoulder. (See Figure 13.)

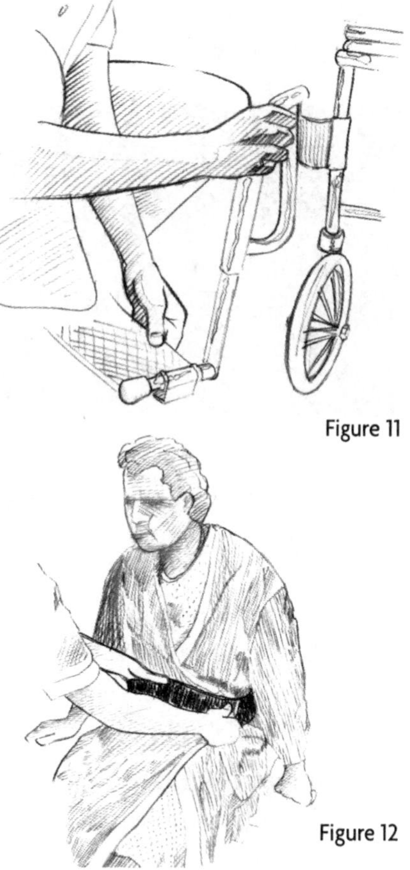

Figure 11

Figure 12

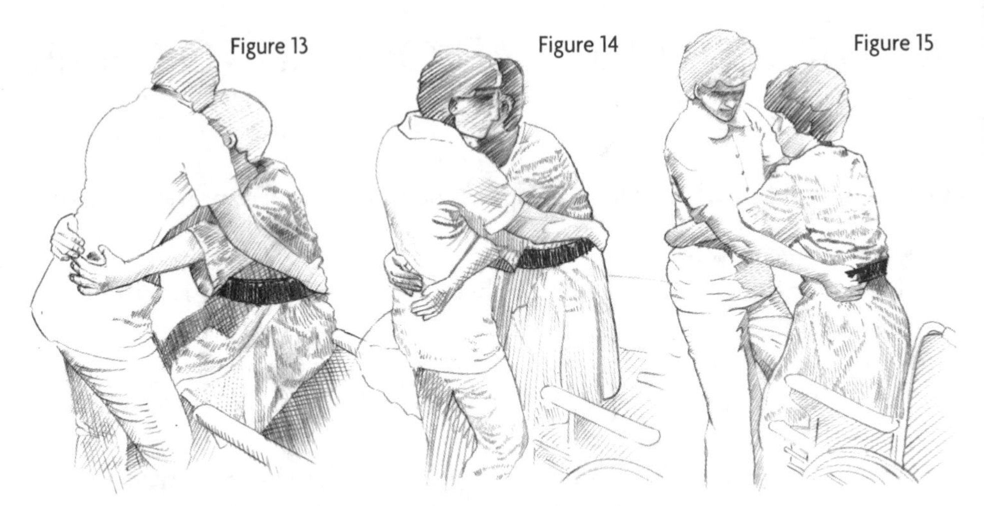


- Rock gently for momentum and count to three. In one continuous movement, stand, pivot, and shuffle together backward until the chair touches the back of the knees, and lower the person into the chair. (See Figures 14 and 15).
- Replace wheelchair armrest and foot pedal.

## IMPORTANT POINTS

- *If the person cannot stand and support their weight, do not attempt this type of move. Ask your home care nurse about availability of a mechanical lift or transfer aide.*
- *An occupational therapist or physiotherapist, if available, may be able to give you advice about how to help with moves. Ask about the availability and use of a transfer belt or other aids.*

# WALKING

■

Although the person may be able to stand and walk, help may still be needed to prevent falls. Some people will be able to use a cane or walking device while others will need support.

**How you can offer care**

The most important thing for you to do is prevent your loved one from falling while walking.

**Prepare the environment:**

- Move all obstacles from your path and any floor covering that may cause a fall.
- Have a chair nearby in case the person needs a rest.
- Make sure both of you are wearing secure non-skid footwear.
- Provide your support on the person's weaker side.
- If a cane is used, have the person hold it on the stronger side. This will keep the weight on the side that can support it.
- Stand beside and slightly behind the person, facing the same direction. When necessary, remind the person to stand tall and to look ahead, not down at the floor.
- Put your arm around the person's waist and use your other hand to hold the person's elbow or hand. Stay close so that your entire body gives support. (See Figure 16.)
- Try using a belt or folded blanket around the person's waist so you can hang on to it to give added support.
- If available, ask a member of your health care team if a transfer belt or walker would make getting around easier.
- Place your arms around the person's lower back or use the waist band, a turning sheet, towel or transfer belt around the back so you support the person.

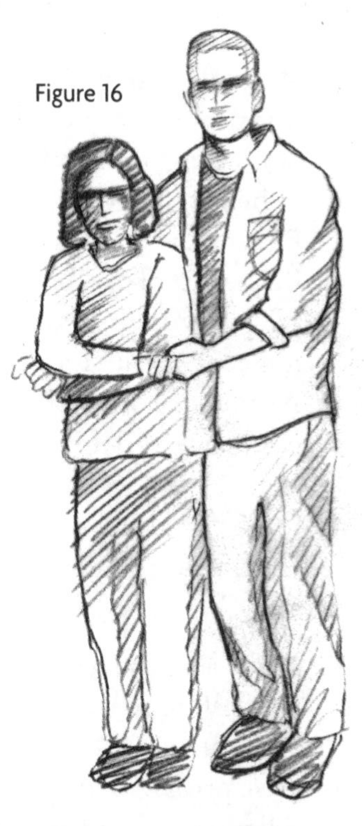

Figure 16

## IMPORTANT POINTS

- *When available, ask an occupational therapist, physiotherapist or home care nurse for advice if you are unsure about helping a person with moving.*
- *Always remember the use of proper body mechanics.*
- *Call for help if:*
  - *you find the person on the floor and suspect an injury.*
  - *you cannot get the person off the floor.*
  - *you have doubts or concerns about moving the person by yourself.*

# TOILETING

■

For some people, the need for help with toileting can be very embarrassing. This is particularly true for someone who is confined to bed.

### What you need to know

- The person may need help to use the toilet, a commode, a urinal or a bedpan depending on mobility.
- When helping with toileting needs, respect your loved one's dignity.
- Be sensitive to the need for privacy.
- Be matter-of-fact about the activity to reduce embarrassment.
- Have environmentally friendly air freshener nearby if scent is tolerated and no scent sensitivities exist.
- As much as possible, ensure that bowel habits follow the same pattern of frequency as before the illness.

## BATHROOM

When the person is able to get up and go to the toilet, offer whatever help is needed. Stay close by.

- Make sure the bathroom floor is dry, the person has non-slip footwear and the path to the toilet is well-lit and free of obstacles.
- Place toilet paper within reach.
- Give privacy if the person can be left alone.
- Allow as much time as needed. The sound of running water might help someone who is having trouble urinating.
- Help with cleaning and wiping-up as needed. Wipe front and back areas separately with clean tissues or cloths.
- Help the person to wash their hands when finished, then wash your own hands.
- Take your time getting back to the bed or chair.
- Check with your nurse or occupational therapist about equipment that makes toileting safer and easier (e.g. a raised toilet seat with side rails).

## COMMODES

Commodes are portable toilets in the shape of a chair. They can be positioned close to the bed of a person who is able to get up but too weak to walk to a bathroom.

- Be sure the brakes are locked on the commode.
- Use the techniques described in *Moving Someone From Bed to Chair* (page 45) to help the person move to and use the commode.
- Let the person do as much as possible. Have toilet paper within reach.
- Once finished, help the person to wash their hands.
- Empty the commode bucket as soon as you have helped the person return to the bed or chair.
- Wash your hands and return the commode to its usual place.

## URINALS

Urinals are small collection bottles that men can use for passing urine. They come in different shapes and sizes and are usually made of plastic. Some are made of metal or moulded cardboard.

- Some men are able to use the urinal lying down, while others prefer sitting on the edge of the bed or standing up. If the person is able and wants to stand, offer support.
- If the person uses the urinal in bed, raise the head of the bed for comfort. Make sure the foot of the bed is down so that urine does not spill out of the urinal.
- Keep the urinal emptied and thoroughly rinsed and clean after every use. This helps prevent spills and offensive odours. Rinsing it with cold water and baking soda will keep odour down.
- Wash your hands after emptying the urinal.
- If the person wants help using the urinal, be sure the penis is placed directly into the urinal and that the urinal is tilted downward.

## BEDPANS

Most people find a bedpan uncomfortable and awkward to use. However, it may be necessary for someone unable to get out of bed.

- You can warm up a bedpan by rinsing it with hot water and then drying it.
- Try some talcum powder on top of the bedpan so it does not stick to the skin.
- If the person is strong enough, bending their knees and placing feet flat on the mattress can help with positioning the bedpan. Help lift the person's bottom while you slide the bedpan under.
- Alternatively, help the person roll away from you. Place an incontinence pad on the mattress, put the bedpan on the mattress where the person's bottom will be and help the person roll back onto the pan. (See Figures 17, 18 and 19.)
- Raise the head of the bed to increase comfort. Have the foot of the bed down so that urine will not pour out by mistake.
- Make sure the person is wiped clean and dry.
- Cover the bedpan before removing it to prevent spilling. Empty it in the toilet and clean it. Rinse with cold water and baking soda to keep it odour free.
- Wash your hands and help the person to wash theirs.

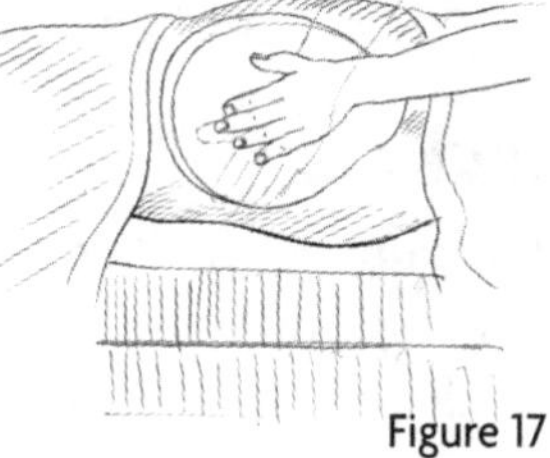

Figure 17

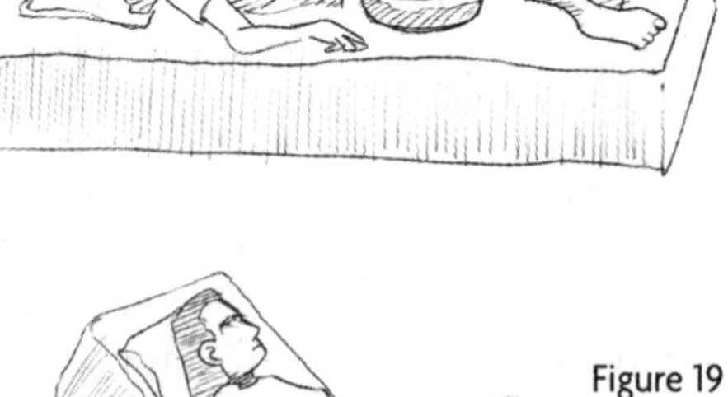

Figure 18

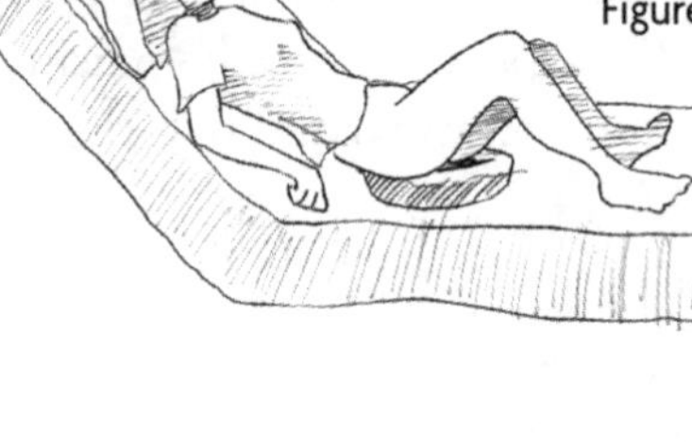

Figure 19

# FOOD AND FLUID CHANGES

■

Enjoying food and drink together is a part of our culture of caring, sharing, continued health and well-being. When a person is newly diagnosed with an advanced progressive illness, it is good to ask for early advice, information and direction on food and nutritional care. Find out if that will be challenged and change as the illness progresses. This helps to better understand how to try to keep optimum nutrition and hydration for as long as possible. It also prepares you to know how an advanced illness can change and reduce appetite, taste, and weight as the end stage of life draws closer.

Depending on the particular progressive illness and symptoms, each situation can be different. Nutritional and fluid concerns need to be addressed, assessed, discussed and understood by you, your loved one, and your health care team.

## NUTRITIONAL SUPPLEMENTS

Food supplement drinks or puddings (commercial or homemade) may help people in certain stages of a progressive illness when they do not want to eat solid food or have difficulty chewing or swallowing. These drinks or puddings provide an easy and convenient source of calories and protein.

### Commercial food supplements

Many commercially prepared supplements can be purchased at your local pharmacy or grocery stores. These include supplements for people who are unable to tolerate lactose or sugar. Alongside brand names such as Ensure™ or Boost™ are generic brands that may cost less. Several products are also available with fibre added. New products and flavours are being developed all the time. To improve the taste, they can be frozen and eaten like ice cream or thickened to make them into a pudding.

### Homemade food supplements

Commercial nutritional supplements are loaded with nutrients. People may or may not like the taste.

- Try offering a power shake, power slushie or smoothie instead.
- A power shake is a milkshake with added nutritional powders that you can buy in pharmacies and health food stores. It is a meal in a glass. You can make the shake in a blender with milk, ice cream and the nutritional powder. Lactose- free products such as Lactaid™ or Rice Dream™ (a non-dairy cream) can also be used. Flavour as the person wishes.
- Power slushies can be used when the person is producing a lot of mucus and you want to avoid dairy products. In a blender, mix the nutritional powder with crushed ice and fruit juice.

## DECREASING APPETITE

As the progressive illness advances, it is difficult to see and understand that someone you love will eat or drink less than usual or not at all. The tendency is to encourage or force them to eat when they are no longer able to do so. Understand that this may cause your loved one more distress, discomfort, and possible increased symptoms such as pain, nausea and vomiting.

- A decreasing appetite is usually normal because the illness is advancing. The body is often unable to tolerate, digest absorb, process or metabolize food as it once did.
- The person may eventually refuse solids, only tolerating liquids or ice chips.
- Noticeable weight loss may be caused by the advanced disease, no matter how much has been eaten.
- A changing sense of taste may alter the enjoyment of food. If it is connected to a treatment or medication, this may be temporary or could become permanent.
- Bitter tastes may develop or food may seem too sweet.
- Some people develop distaste for meat, or for certain textures and smells of food.
- Even when eating and drinking is reduced, attention is still needed to ensure regular bowel patterns and interventions.

### How you can offer comfort and care

Aim to understand your loved one's point of view and find realistic ways to offer nourishing foods if tolerated.

Try to make a pleasant, quiet and peaceful eating environment. For instance, remove bedpans or commodes and clutter from the area. Keep cooking smells and noises as far away as you can manage.

- Check that the mouth has no sores as this can also lower food and fluid intake.
- Try new spices and flavourings for foods. Tastes often change during illness.
- Avoid highly seasoned or salty foods.
- Add sauces and gravies to dry food.
- Flavour food with sugar, basil, seasonings, lemon juice or mint.
- Add fruit and juice to milkshakes, custards, ice cream and puddings.
- Marinate meat in soya sauce, sweet juices or sweet wines.
- Try alternative high protein foods such as eggs, poultry or fish with someone who has developed a dislike of meat.
- Offer high protein, high calorie snacks such as eggnogs, cream soups and ice cream.
- Choose foods that are soft and easy to eat.
- Avoid foods that have similar textures to the foods the person dislikes.
- Try serving water, tea or soft drinks to take a strange taste away. Sometimes adding citrus juices such as lemon to foods can make a taste more normal.
- Increase or decrease the sweetness of foods if the person finds this improves flavours.
- Vary food colour and use garnishes to make food attractive.
- Serve favourite foods in very small portions on small attractive plates, offering them five or six times a day.
- Plan small, frequent meals at times when the person has least pain or other symptoms and is well rested.
- Have dentures relined or try a product such as Polygrip™ if they are loose.
- Tell your home care nurse if nausea is a problem, as medications can be tried.
- Make breakfast a high nourishing meal, as appetite tends to reduce as the day progresses.
- Try a glass of beer or wine to stimulate the appetite unless this is not recommended by the doctor.
- Encourage the person to eat food low in fat, to chew slowly and pause occasionally during the meal to avoid feeling full too quickly.
- Freshen and clean the person's mouth before and after eating.

- Make meal time a social occasion. Someone who is not able to go to the table may enjoy having you sit at the bedside and perhaps sharing a meal there.
- Eat in a calm and relaxed atmosphere. Dimmed lights and favorite music might help.
- Eliminate the metallic taste in food by cooking in glass pots and using plastic utensils.
- Offer cold plates such as cottage cheese and fruit plates if the smell of food is a problem.
- To clear the taste buds, clean and rinse the person's mouth before and after eating.

## GIVING HELP WITH EATING

■

The very act of eating can present challenges. Along with having no appetite, the ill person may not even have energy to eat.

### How you can offer comfort and care

You can do some things to make it easier for your loved one to try to eat.

- Practice feeding someone with a friend or family member. Switch roles so you are aware of both sides of the feeding experience.
- Encourage the person to rest after meals. Keep the head of the bed elevated to help digestion.
- Adjust the diet if the person can no longer wear dentures. Soft foods or small bite-size portions of meat, softened with gravy, are ideal.
- Keep in mind that the person may not remember to eat. Offer small snacks throughout the day.
- Assess the person's ability to chew and swallow before you serve solid foods. For someone who can swallow but cannot chew, a puree or pudding would be most effective. For someone who can chew, keep food pieces small so less energy is needed to eat.
- Give liquids and solids separately.
- Give finger foods if the person prefers or can only eat with fingers. This will help to maintain a level of independence.
- Be sure that the person's head is well supported and upright when eating or being fed.
- Use bibs or large napkins when necessary to help keep clothing and bedding clean.

- Use a spoon instead of a fork when you are feeding someone. This prevents accidental stabs with a fork prong. Also, a long-handled spoon will help you place the food far enough into the mouth.
- Offer small spoonfuls and place food at the front of the mouth. Wait until the last spoonful is swallowed before offering the next.
- If nausea is a problem, be prepared. Keep a small basin or bowl close by, as vomiting can happen very suddenly.

## IMPORTANT POINTS

- *Ask your doctor, pharmacist or home care nurse if any medications may be of benefit to try to improve appetite.*
- *Tell your home care nurse if nausea, dry or sore mouth, or problems swallowing are affecting the person's eating.*
- *If the person coughs or chokes frequently when eating or drinking, stop the feeding immediately. Ask your home care nurse or doctor to do a swallowing assessment and let you know if and when it is safe to continue to try feeding.*
- *Never force a person to eat or drink.*

Often as illness progresses to the final stage, your loved one will rest and sleep more, having little or no appetite or ability to swallow. This is an even more special time. Concentrate now on being totally present, spending quality time and providing comfort through gentle touch and care.

## REDUCED FLUID INTAKE

Fluids usually help to flush out a healthy body of waste products and keep cells and skin well hydrated. If advancing illness means your loved one is no longer able or wishes to drink much fluid, dehydration may occur. This condition means there is not enough normal body fluid to be regularly absorbed. This may be caused by many reasons, such as progression of the illness, symptoms such as nausea and vomiting, constipation, and confusion. Whether an intervention to replace the fluid will be beneficial will depend on the cause.

Just as with reduced appetite, reduced fluid intake needs to be addressed, assessed, discussed and understood by your loved one, you and your health care team.

## How you can offer comfort and care

- Always have fluids close at hand. These include water, juice, coffee, tea, ice chips, broths and nutritional supplements. Water flavoured with lemon juice is refreshing.
- Change the fluids often to keep them fresh.
- Ice chips or popsicles are excellent ways to give fluids. Also, they help to keep the mouth moist and feeling fresh.
- Raise the person's head when helping to drink. Use a few pillows or gently support the base of the head with your hand. It is almost impossible to drink when lying flat.
- Ask your loved one to take small sips and not big gulps to help prevent choking.
- Use a short straw that bends if the person is strong enough to draw up the liquid through it.
- If lips no longer fit tightly around the rim of a glass, try a spill-free thermos bottle or cup to make drinking easier.
- Use a gentle reminder if the person forgets to swallow. Sometimes softly stroking the side of the throat will help to stimulate swallowing.
- The person can swallow but finds it difficult. After assessment by the health care team, it may be suggested that you offer fluids that are somewhat thick and easier to swallow such as milkshakes and applesauce.
- Each person's advanced illness and symptoms are unique. Talking with your doctor and home care nurse about what is happening, what to expect and the pros and cons of artificial hydration options is very important.

- If the person is not drinking because of symptoms causing problems that artificial fluids may help, an intervention called hypodermoclysis may be considered. Hypodermoclysis puts fluid into body tissues using a small subcutaneous needle (placed just under the skin). It is attached to a plastic tube and a bag of water. Check with your doctor and home care nurse to see if this method would suit the illness and symptoms and whether it is used in your community. If so, your home care nurse can set it up and give you a copy of the information and guidelines to start and maintain it as needed. Deciding whether to continue will depend on whether it relieves symptoms, or causes others such as increased fluid retention and swelling, nausea and vomiting, increased secretions and congestion.

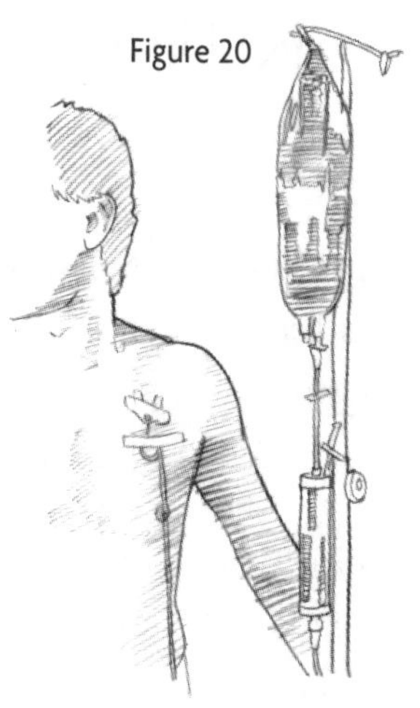
Figure 20

## IMPORTANT POINTS

- *As your loved one's condition advances to the final stage it is often more important to focus on trying to drink some liquids to keep the mouth moist, rather than forcing eating.*
- *Intervention aimed at reducing dehydration must consider the cause of the symptom, the disease course, patient/family values and shared goals of care.*
- *Withdrawing from taking food and fluid is a common, natural part of the dying process.*
- *Most dying people do not indicate they feel thirst or hunger as death approaches.*
- *Giving food and fluids by artificial means (e.g., intravenously or subcutaneously) in the end stage of illness does not necessarily prolong life or improve its quality.*
- *Artificial hydration does not provide nutrition.*
- *Hydration may not prevent or improve thirst or relieve a dry mouth.*
- *Caring support for your loved one includes frequent mouth care, ice chips, oral mist, and artificial saliva to relieve a dry mouth.*

*One 2013 website resource, www.virtualhospice.ca, may help in better understanding food and fluid changes. Search this site for more information on decreased food and fluids, lack of appetite, loss of weight, and dehydration.*

# NUTRITIONAL SUPPLEMENT RECIPES

■

**HIGH PROTEIN MILK**
*(180 calories, 15 grams protein)*

**Blend:** 1 cup milk (250 mL)
¼ cup skim milk powder (50 mL)

**MILKSHAKE** *(380 calories, 20 grams protein)*

**Blend:** 1 cup high protein milk (250 mL)
¾ cup ice cream (200 mL)

**PEANUT BUTTER SHAKE**
*(510 calories, 20 grams protein)*

**Blend:** ¾ cup ice cream (200 mL)
½ cup milk (125 mL)
¼ cup skim milk powder (50 mL)
2 Tbsp. peanut butter (30 mL)

**FRUIT SHAKE** *(350 calories)*

**Blend:** ½ cup whole milk
½ cup canned peaches or other fruits
1 cup vanilla ice cream

**STRAWBERRY DELIGHT**
*(765 calories, 20 grams protein)*

**Blend:** 1 cup ice cream (250 mL)
¾ cup milk (200 mL)
¾ cup half and half cream (200 mL)
¼ cup skim milk powder (50 mL)
2 Tbsp. strawberry jam (30 mL)

**YOGURT SHAKE** *(290 calories, 15 grams protein)*

**Blend:** ¾ cup plain yogurt (200 mL)
¼ cup skim milk powder (50 mL)
½ cup apple juice (125 mL)
1 Tbsp. sugar or honey (15 mL)

**SUPER PUDDING**
*(1,065 calories, 35 grams protein)*

**Blend:** 1 pkg. (4-½ oz., 113 grams) instant pudding
2 cups milk (500 mL)
2 Tbsp. oil (30 mL)
¾ cup skim milk powder (200 mL)

**SOUP PLUS** *(295 calories, 20 grams protein)*

**Blend:** 1 cup cream soup (250 mL)
2 oz. cooked meat or poultry (50 grams)
2 Tbsp. skim milk powder (50 mL)

# LIQUID FEEDINGS

■

These recipes can be useful if the person has problems swallowing or chewing solid food.

**HOT BLENDER** *(Yield: 6 - 6 oz. servings, 155 calories per serving)*

1 cup cooked meat (chopped fine) or canned baby food meat

1 cup cooked carrots or other vegetables

2 small cooked potatoes

2 cups whole milk

1 cup canned or home-made cream soup

Blend until smooth and heat.

**COLD BLENDER** *(Yield: 6 - 6 oz. servings, 265 calories per serving)*

2 cups ice cream and add

2 ½ cups whole milk

1 cup cereal cream

½ cup sugar

Blend and add syrup or flavour if desired

## IMPORTANT POINTS

*Seek dietetic guidance when considering and using supplements.*
*To safely use homemade supplements:*

- *keep them refrigerated.*
- *discard after 24 hours in the fridge, or two hours at room temperature.*

*Follow these instructions carefully as these supplements spoil easily.*

# MEDICATIONS

■

Your attention to the proper care and use of medications will help increase the benefits they offer.

### What you need to know

Your loved one may have many medications prescribed. It is essential that they be handled carefully and accurately. If the person is not able to do this alone, you can help in several ways.

- Keeping records of medications is very important, especially when regular doses of pain relief are being given. A good recording system will help you keep organized.
- A chart showing a list of medications, the doses and when each is taken will help the doctor know if there is a need to change the drug or the dose. (see Appendix III Home Medication Schedule, page 151).
- Heat and light can change the chemical composition of some medicines.
- Most medications are best stored in a cool, dark place.
- Some medications must be kept in the refrigerator. Make sure they will not freeze and that children cannot get at them.
- Many medications have an expiry date. If a drug is too old to use, talk to your home care nurse about proper disposal of it.
- Medications should be kept in a safe place out of the reach of children or anyone who might take them accidentally.
- Do not talk in public about the medications you have in your home. Keep them in a secure place out of sight. There is always a risk that someone may try breaking in to steal them.

## IMPORTANT POINTS ABOUT ANY METHOD OF GIVING MEDICATION

- *Never try to give oral medications to someone who is asleep or unconscious.*
- *Use the right medicine, in the right amount, at the right time. Administer the medication by the correct method liquids, tablets, drops, ointment, sprays, suppositories, or injections.*
- *If medications are over-the-counter products or are ordered by more than one doctor, ask your doctor or pharmacist if they can be safely taken together.*
- *Check with your home care nurse or pharmacist if you notice sudden behaviour changes, hallucinations or other mild or severe reactions.*
- *Keep medications out of the reach of a person who is confused.*
- *If the person is using products from a health food store or over the counter remedies, tell your doctor or pharmacist so you avoid the risk of conflicts. For instance, some herbs may interfere with prescribed medications.*
- *Alert the health care professionals to any allergies.*
- *Call for help if a needle site becomes red, swollen, leaks, bleeds or causes discomfort.*
- *When you get a prescription filled, ask about side effects so you know what to expect. Be sure the medication is safe with other drugs being used. (Bring a list of those other medications with you.)*
- *Find out if any food or drinks (such as alcohol) might interfere with the benefits of the drug.*

### How you can offer care

Follow the instructions for proper use of medications and do not hesitate to ask for advice if you are not sure.

- Discuss with your home care nurse and pharmacist how you can set up a schedule for the medications and help the person take them properly.
- Try to use the same pharmacist all the time. That person will understand your situation and be in a better position to answer your questions.
- Remember that it might take a few days to get a new supply of a prescription drug. Keep track of how much you have left of any medication and how long it will last.
- Keep all your stock of medication in one place.
- Have someone in charge of keeping track of what is needed. Be sure to order more before the present supply runs out.

- It is very easy to mix up medications, especially when several different ones are being used.
- Try to organize the way you store drugs so it is easy to tell them apart.
- Keep a medication chart nearby for quick checking.
- Try colour coding – mark each label with a coloured dot, then put a matching dot beside the medication's name on a chart. This will help you be sure you are giving the right one.
- Check each medication twice as you are preparing it. Read the label when you pick up the container and again when you are finished preparation to be sure it is the correct one.
- Ask your pharmacist or home care nurse about a medication dispenser to help organize a long list of drugs to be taken. These dispensers are called dosettes. Your pharmacist may also be able to help organize the medications into groupings contained in packaging called blister or bubble packs. (See Figure 21.)

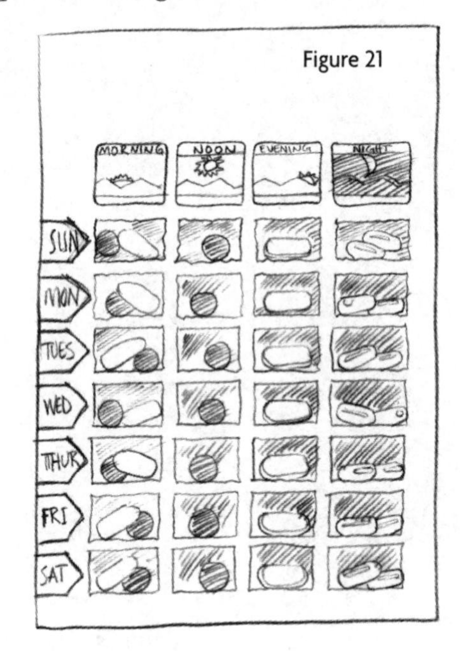

Figure 21

## GIVING MEDICATIONS BY MOUTH

Medications given by mouth are also called oral medications. They include anything that is swallowed – pills, capsules, tablets, lozenges, syrups and elixirs. Oral medications are the safest and easiest way to get a medication into the body.

- Wash your hands before you handle the medication.
- Most oral medications are meant to be swallowed right away.
- Some oral medications such as lozenges are sucked or chewed. Lozenges should not be swallowed whole.
- For pills, capsules or tablets, offer a glass of water or juice to help the person swallow. Suggest a sip of fluid before taking the pill to lubricate the mouth and help swallowing. Avoid milk unless you have been told the medication should be taken this way.
- Help the person sit up or raise the head to make swallowing easier. Never give an oral medication to someone who is lying down as this could lead to choking.
- Some medicines are hard on the stomach. Do not give oral medications on an empty stomach unless that is what the instructions say to do. Check the labels on the package or bottle and do what they say.
- Be sure a medication has been swallowed before you record it on the medication chart.
- If the person is having trouble swallowing pills, try some of these tips:
    - Offer some water first to moisten the throat, place pills at the back of the tongue and follow with more water. Try to encourage the person to relax the throat while swallowing.
    - Mix pills in applesauce, jam, ice cream, sherbet or pudding – anything that has substance enough to carry the pills down the throat. Some pills can be crushed and then mixed – check which ones can be crushed with your doctor or pharmacist first.
    - Small pills can be put into a gelatin capsule by your pharmacist, and swallowed together in one capsule instead of separately.
    - Ask your pharmacist if the medication comes in a liquid form. If so, talk to your doctor about changing the prescription.
    - If the person is taking a liquid medication and does not like the taste, keep the bottle in the refrigerator or disguise the taste with another liquid like pop, juice or milk. Use different liquids so the bad taste does not become associated with any one drink.

- If the person is still not able to swallow the medications, ask your pharmacist or doctor about alternative methods such as a suppository or skin patch. It is important that the medication schedule not be interrupted.
- If the person is having side effects or the medication is not working the way you expected, talk with your home care nurse.

## GIVING MEDICATIONS BY SUPPOSITORY

A suppository is a medication moulded into a small solid shape that can be put into the rectum. This route is a useful alternative when medications cannot be given by mouth. Suppositories are used most often to relieve pain, constipation, nausea, vomiting or fever.

- Most suppositories are kept in the refrigerator, but do not use one directly from there. It will be cold and could be uncomfortable. Let it warm up first.
- To give a suppository, you need latex gloves and a lubricant such as K-Y Jelly™. Collect everything you need before you begin.
- Help the person into a position that will make it easy to insert the suppository.
- The best position is lying on the left side, with the upper leg bent forward.
- Put on the glove and lubricate the suppository. If you do not have a lubricant, wetting the suppository will make it easier to insert.
- Ask the person to take a deep breath and try to relax the muscles around the anus. Slow, rhythmic deep breathing will help to relax muscles.
- Spread the buttocks with one hand to expose the anus. Then, with the other hand, slide the suppository inside about two inches.
- The suppository may trigger the urge to have a bowel movement, but encourage the person to hold on. The suppository needs 10 to 15 minutes to dissolve.

## GIVING MEDICATIONS ABSORBED THROUGH THE SKIN (TRANSDERMAL)

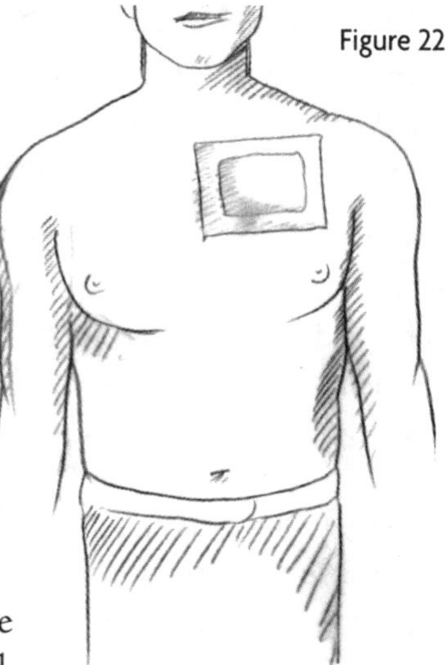

Figure 22

Some medications are absorbed through the skin. Most come as creams or ointments that are put on the skin. Some come as patches that are put on the skin and taped in place, or have their own adhesive.

- With creams and ointments, it may be important to wear gloves so that you do not come into contact with the medication. Ask your pharmacist.
- When putting on medication patches:
  - Select a clean, dry area of skin on the front or back, above the waist. (The medication is absorbed best at this location).

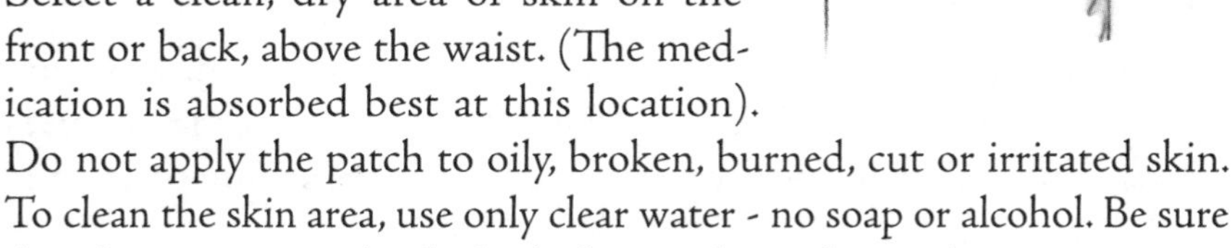

    Do not apply the patch to oily, broken, burned, cut or irritated skin. To clean the skin area, use only clear water - no soap or alcohol. Be sure that the area is completely dry before applying the patch.
  - Clip a hairy area with scissors but do not shave it.
  - Remove the skin patch from its protective pouch and peel off the strip.
  - Try not to touch the sticky side.
  - Put the sticky side against the skin.
  - Press the patch firmly for about 10 to 20 seconds with the palm of your hand. Be sure that the edges stick to the person's skin.
  - Tape the patch in place with paper if it is not self-adhesive. Tape the top, sides and bottom so the patch looks like it has a frame around it. (See Figure 22.)
  - Wash your hands.
- Apply each new patch to a different skin area to avoid irritation. Remove the old patch before applying another one.
- If the patch comes off accidentally or the skin under the patch becomes irritated, replace it with a new one in a different area. Be sure the new skin area is clean and dry.
- Make a written schedule of when patches should be changed.
- Some people write a date directly onto the patch as it is easy to lose track of when it was applied.
- Dispose of used and leftover unused patches immediately. The procedure for disposal varies across the province, so ask your home care nurse how it is done in your community.

## GIVING SUBCUTANEOUS MEDICATIONS

Subcutaneous means 'just under the skin.' For a subcutaneous injection, a tiny needle is placed under the skin (subcutaneous tissue). This needle is left in place and taped securely for repeated use.

Most medications for controlling symptoms can be given by subcutaneous injections rather than by intravenous (IV). The subcutaneous method is easier, safer and does not restrict the person's movement as an IV would. An IV may be needed if the person needs IV antibiotics or blood products, but this is seldom necessary to keep a person comfortable at home

### What you need to know

If your loved one is not able to take medications by mouth, a subcutaneous injection may be used.

- If you want to learn how to start a subcutaneous needle, the home care nurse will teach you. Ask the nurse to leave a copy of the instructions for inserting and removing the subcutaneous needle, and preparing and giving the injection.
- Whether or not you choose to insert the subcutaneous needle, the home care nurse will start it and will help you maintain this treatment.
- The needle is very small. It may sting when first inserted but should not cause any further pain.
- The needle is usually put into the abdomen or chest but can also be placed in the thigh, upper arm or back.
- The needle has a tube. A rubber stopper through which medication is given can be attached to the tube. (See Figure 23.)

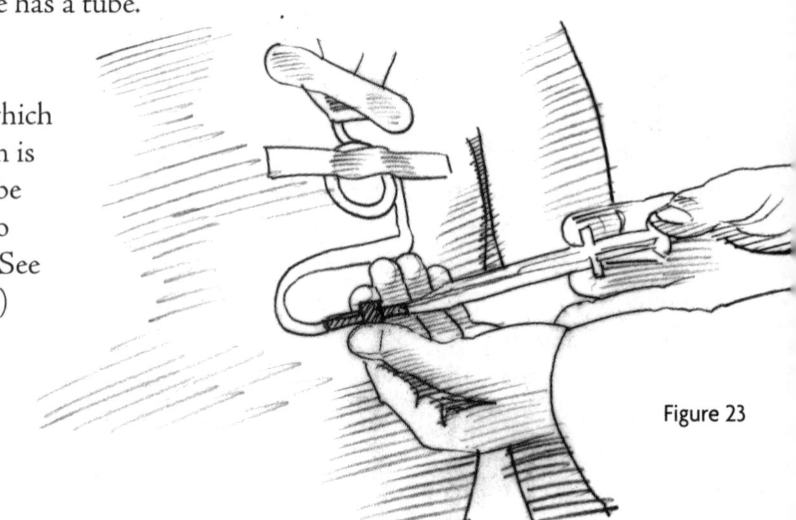

Figure 23

- Your home care nurse may pre-load medication into a syringe and ask you to give it because of the timing or frequency of the dose. This may mean giving the medication at scheduled times or when requested by the person.
- Your home care nurse will show you how to wipe the rubber stopper with an alcohol swab and inject the medication.
- Another way of giving medications is to attach a pump that will include a small container of medication. There are different types of pumps. The person may be able to self-administer the medication using a pump. There are also computerized pumps that can be set to administer the medication continuously. (See Figures 24 and 25.)

Figure 24

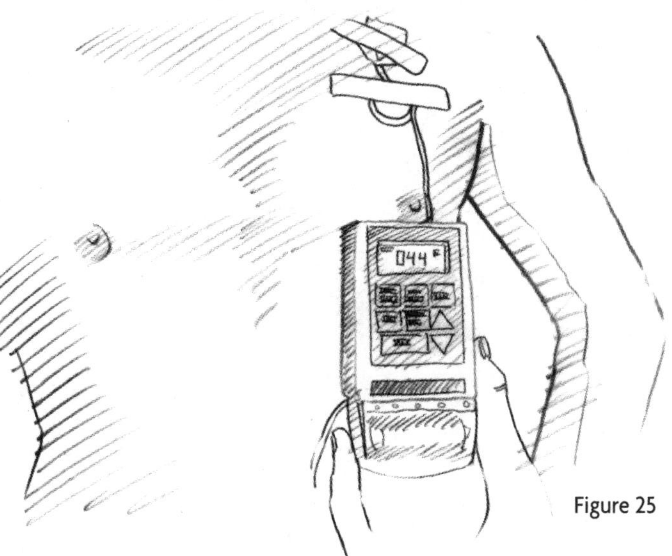

Figure 25

- The pump may be provided through the hospital, or you may need to rent it. Your home care nurse can let you know which system is used in your community, and can help you organize it.
- A subcutaneous needle is usually left in place between four to seven days, depending on the type of medication going in. However, some sites last longer. Let the home care nurse know if a site becomes red or swollen.

### How you can offer comfort

- Explain the reason for the subcutaneous needle, saying that it is important that medications use continues, especially if swallowing medication has become difficult.
- Reassure the person that once the needle is inserted, there should be minimal further discomfort.

CHAPTER

# 3

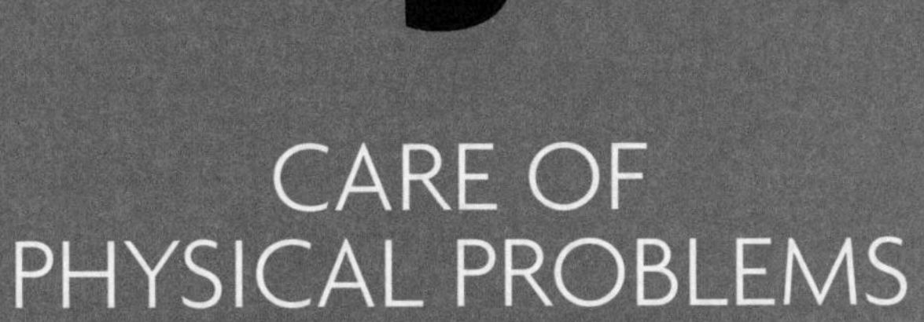

# CARE OF PHYSICAL PROBLEMS

# PAIN

■

When someone complains of physical pain, it is usually at a particular location in the body. However, a general feeling of not being well is sometimes experienced and described as pain or discomfort.

## WHAT YOU NEED TO KNOW

To help someone in pain, it is important to assess the pain. It is also important to know that people explain and express pain in different ways. Pain can be more than just physical. It can also be emotional, social, spiritual, and many other different elements that are often described as "total pain."

### Points to Remember:

- Assessing pain is an ongoing process. You need to ask and know as much as you can about the person's pain at any given time.
- The feeling of pain may be worse if the person is having other physical symptoms such as nausea.
- Feelings such as worry, fear, boredom and loneliness may make the experience of pain worse. It is better to first explore and attend to these particular needs, and not just automatically increase pain medications.
- Understanding more about the pain will help you to provide comfort and let you know if the help you are giving is working.

### How you can offer comfort and care

No one is more expert about the pain than the person who is feeling it. If the person you are caring for complains of pain, believe it. Even if there is no complaint, you need to be observant. Ask about any signs of discomfort you see.

The experience of pain is different for each person. After asking the following questions, you can provide the doctor or home care nurse with information that can help address and take care of the pain. As there may be more than one physical pain, ask the same questions in relation to each pain.

- Where is the pain? Is it one particular place or is it all over?
- Can you point to where the pain is? Is it deep inside or on the surface? Is there more than one type of pain?"
- When did the pain begin – an hour ago, yesterday, or months ago?
- How often does the pain occur?
- How long does the pain last – minutes, hours? Does it come and go, or is it constant?
- What does the pain feel like? Ask the person to describe it. Provide examples of words to use – stabbing, burning, aching, throbbing, piercing.
- How much does it hurt? It often helps to ask the person to rate their pain on a scale from zero to 10, where zero is no pain and 10 is the worst yet.
- What could have started the pain – was it movement, eating, pressure, the way the person was lying or sitting?
- What makes the pain go away – rest, massage, movement, meditation, distraction, medication?
- To what degree is the pain limiting normal activities?
- What other symptoms are present?
- The ongoing use of a pain rating scale can give valuable information about the pain experience over time. A rating scale used every day can help evaluate pain. This information can be put on a graph. From the graphed results, your home care nurse can help you decide if you should contact the doctor for a change of medication. (see Appendix IV Symptom Assessment Scale, page 152)., and the *Wong-Baker Pain Rating Scale,* below).

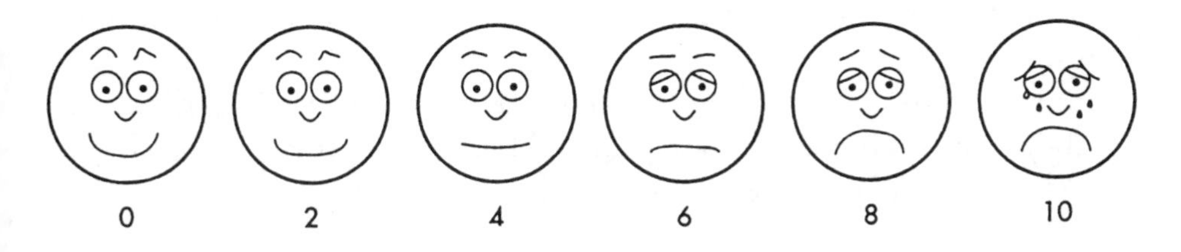

## IMPORTANT POINTS

**Ask for help if:**

- *A new pain occurs - different from the person's usual pain.*
- *Pain continues after you have given three breakthrough doses in 24 hours.* (See information on 'breakthrough' in next section, *Managing Pain with Medications*)
- *There is a rapid increase in the intensity of the pain.*
- *There is sudden acute pain.*
- *You notice sudden confusion (see* Confusion, *page 76).*

# MANAGING PAIN WITH MEDICATIONS

■

Someone who has constant pain needs regular pain medication to control it.

**What you need to know**

- The goal of pain management is to keep someone alert, with the pain under control as much as possible. It takes time and testing to arrive at the exact combination of medications that will keep a person feeling more comfortable. You can shorten this process by regularly recording positive or negative effects of a new medication and talking to the home care nurse and doctor about the results.
- A record of the pain and of regular scheduled pain medication and breakthrough doses will help the doctor adjust the dose (see Pain, page 70).

## WORLD HEALTH ORGANIZATION ANALGESIC LADDER

- Medications that provide relief from pain are called analgesics. Two basic groups of analgesics are opioids and non-opioids.
- Opioids are analgesics defined by the Canadian Narcotic Control Act as controlled substances. (Although the word narcotic is often used for these medications, the proper word is opioid.) They are used for moderate to severe pain.
- Non-opioids are probably the most commonly used medications. They include products to ease pain and lower fever. They are usually prescribed for mild to moderate pain.

## How you can offer comfort and care

Some basic guidelines apply to the use of any pain relief medication.

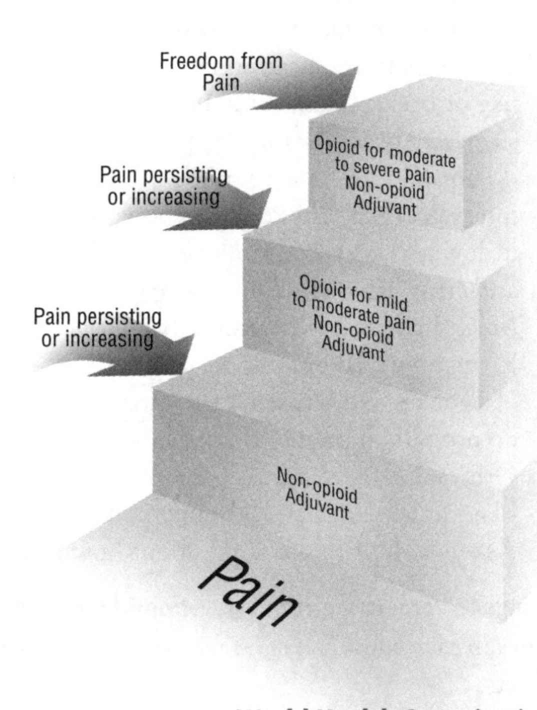


**World Health Organization Analgesic Ladder**

- When pain is constant, give the medication on schedule even if there is no pain at the time. This helps make sure the pain stays away. Once the pain returns, it becomes more difficult to control. (Using a timer can help you keep track of the schedule for pain medication.)
- Plan to give physical care after a medication has started to work in order to reduce discomfort. Most pain medications take effect within approximately 30-40 minutes. This is useful to know, especially if you must change a dressing or move a person around more in bed.
- When taken regularly, pain medication is just as effective taken by mouth as by injection. Alternative routes such as injections, suppositories or patches are considered when the person cannot take or tolerate medication by mouth.

## Things to remember about opioid pain medicines

- Short-acting opioids require a dose every three to four hours to keep a person in constant pain more comfortable. If the person is not on long-acting opioids, set an alarm to wake yourself up for night time doses. Otherwise the person will wake up in pain. It is then more difficult to catch up to control the pain.
- Keep track of pain relief. If the person has been on a stable dose of pain medication for three to four days, the doctor can consider prescribing a longer acting opioid. Some of these long acting opioids last 12 hours or 24 hours. One is available as a patch that lasts for three days. A person's pain must first be under control on short acting opioids for the long acting form to work well.

- Sometimes pain will 'breakthrough' even when it should be controlled by medication. For example, a person may feel mild or even severe pain a few hours before the next scheduled dose. When this happens, a 'breakthrough' dose of pain medication is often ordered. Guidelines for the frequency of use of breakthrough medication vary. Ask your home care nurse for the suggested breakthrough frequency guideline in your area. Definitely tell your doctor and home care nurse if breakthrough medication, given at hourly intervals three times or more over 24 hours, does not relieve the pain. Write it down to keep track of every breakthrough medication the person takes, and why. This helps the doctor adjust the regular dose. (see Appendix V Breakthrough Medication Chart, page 153).
- Remember that opioids are potent medications and should be kept safely out of sight and out of reach of children and others. As with any other medication, do not talk in public about the fact that you have these drugs in your home. Otherwise, there is a risk someone may try to steal them.
- Have at least a one-week supply of opioid medications on hand.
- Ask your home care nurse about how to dispose of unused opioids.

### Things to remember about non-opioid pain medications

You can take some steps to make pain relief more effective and reduce unwanted effects.

- Take medications as directed on the packaging or by your health care provider.
- Unless you are told otherwise, offer the medication with food to lessen stomach upset.
- Acetaminophen (Tylenol™) can be taken on an empty stomach to improve the way it is absorbed.
- Watch for signs of bleeding or bruising, as some of these medications can affect the blood's clotting.

# POSSIBLE SIDE EFFECTS OR COMPLICATIONS OF OPIOIDS

■

## DROWSINESS

When a new opioid medication is given for the first time, it may initially make that person extra sleepy for a few days. Remember that the person may also be tired from exhaustion and lack of sleep due to pain, and now needs to catch up on sleep.

Let the person catnap whenever desired. Just be sure you are able to rouse the person. In the final days or hours of their illness, this may not be possible. Talk more with your health team to get advice.

## NAUSEA AND VOMITING

When first used, strong opioids can cause queasiness or even make a person throw up. These problems usually disappear in a few days.

- Nausea and vomiting can also be an effect of other medications the person is taking or a result of the illness itself.
- Encourage resting in bed for the first hour or so after taking pain medication.
- Remind the person that pain can also cause nausea and vomiting. If this is the case, the pain medication may also help relieve the nausea and vomiting.
- Ask the home care nurse and doctor about an anti-nausea medication to be taken for three or four days when starting a new opioid or having an opioid dose increase (see Nausea and Vomiting, page 94).

## CONSTIPATION

Opioids slow down the gut. Constipation can be an ongoing problem for someone taking regular opioid medications.

- Anyone taking opioids should also be taking a bowel stimulant and a laxative to prevent constipation (see Constipation, page 87).
- Tell your home care nurse immediately if there is any change in regular bowel routine.

## CONFUSION

A person who is taking pain medications, especially opioids, may feel a little confused. Some people may even have hallucinations, although this is an unusual response.

If confusion occurs, tell your home care nurse. Lower doses of the opioid medication or changing to another opioid type may be recommended. In addition, other aspects of the disease may be causing the confusion and will need to be assessed at the same time.

## MYOCLONUS

This is a twitching or spasm of the muscles that the person cannot control.

- Myoclonus is a similar feeling to the one that can occur when you are just about asleep and suddenly jump awake.
- It is not an unusual response to some medications. The twitching is not related at all to a convulsion.
- Tell your home care nurse if myoclonus is happening.

## ADDICTION VERSUS PHYSICAL DEPENDENCE

There is a difference between addiction and physical dependence. Physical dependence is the body's need to relieve constant physical pain by taking medication regularly to maintain the effect. When the medication is stopped, the body will experience symptoms of withdrawal. Addiction is what some people refer to as psychological dependence – there is no physical need to feel a 'high' from the medication or unwillingness to be without the sensation it gives.

One of the greatest myths about pain management is that people who are taking medications for pain become addicted to them. People do not become addicted to pain medications that are needed for pain and used correctly.

Research has shown that less than one per cent of hospitalized patients receiving opioids for pain will become addicted.

## TOLERANCE

Many people taking pain medication will usually need a higher dose over time because the body develops a tolerance for it. The dose of an opioid can be increased as much as necessary by the doctor in order to relieve pain.

## OPIOID TOXICITY

All the food, water or medications that you take into your body are either useable or waste. Your liver does the job of breaking the parts down and your lungs, bowels and kidneys get rid of the waste. Someone who is on high doses or long term opioid pain relief, or has kidney problems, may have wastes from the medication build up in the body. This is called opioid toxicity.

### What you should know

With opioid toxicity, the person has very marked behaviour changes. If your loved one is using opioids for pain relief, be aware of the signs that indicate problems.

- Delirium or confusion may be seen in the form of:
    - agitation.
    - bad dreams, nightmares.
    - decreased level of consciousness, drowsiness.
    - confusion about time and place.
    - hallucinations (seeing, feeling or hearing things that are not real).
    - moaning and rambling speech.
    - reduced concentration.
    - restlessness.
    - short term memory difficulty.
    - sleeping during the day and waking during the night.
    - jerking or seizure-like movements of limbs or face muscles.
    - seizures.
    - pain when touched in a way not expected to cause pain.
- If you notice any of these changes, tell your home care nurse.
- A member of your health care team may ask questions to check the person's memory and recognition, so that early signs of this complication can be identified.

**What may be done**

- If the person is able to tolerate increased fluid intake or fluid supplementation, the goal would be to increase hydration by mouth so that the kidneys can flush out the toxins. If drinking more fluids is not possible, the team may consider using artificial fluids (through a vein or skin) to flush them out.
- The doctor may switch opioids. Different opioids make different wastes. By switching from one kind to another, the body can continue to get rid of the wastes.
- If the kidneys are not working properly, the doctor may lower the dose of opioid.
- The doctor may order a medication to control hallucinations, nightmares or agitation until the body gets rid of the wastes.

**IMPORTANT POINTS**

*Call for help if you see any of the signs of opioid toxicity.*

# OTHER WAYS TO MANAGE PAIN RELIEF

■

Pain control can sometimes be successfully managed using other methods.

## TENS (TRANSCUTANEOUS NERVE STIMULATION)

This technique involves using a small electronic device using electrode placements to send weak electric pulses through the skin to the underlying nerves. It is thought that the mild electrical activity helps to relieve pain. Your home care nurse can tell you if it might help and if it is available in your community.

- The placing of the electrodes depends on the area and type of pain. A physiotherapist or other member of the health care team who is trained in TENS can teach you where to put the electrodes and how to use the TENS machine.
- The electrodes should not be placed inside an area where radiation is presently being given. As well, avoid these areas for 10 to 14 days after radiation treatment is completed.
- TENS should not be used over sinuses, eyes and ears.
- Do not use TENS on anyone with a pacemaker.
- TENS should not be used near the heart.
- TENS should not be placed on sore, swollen, infected or unhealthy skin.

### OTHER FORMS OF NON-MEDICATION PAIN RELIEF

Some complementary therapies can help distract from pain and may offer pain relief (see Complementary Care, page 101).

- For nerve pain, a local anesthetic can be injected around nerves to block pain that is occurring in one area. The results may be temporary or long lasting.
- Acupuncture is an ancient Chinese treatment that uses sterile needles placed at specific places in the body to relieve pain.
- Radiation can be used to shrink tumours to reduce a person's pain and other symptoms.

## SKIN PROBLEMS

■

### ITCHING

Itching is an unpleasant sensation that causes a desire to scratch or rub the skin. Common causes of itching during a progressive illness include dry skin, allergies, side effects of medications, chemotherapy, or radiation therapy and tumour growth.

#### What you could expect

A terminal illness can cause many changes in the skin. Some of these changes can be very uncomfortable and may lead to restlessness, anxiety, skin sores and infection.

- Skin may be dry, red, rough, and flaky.
- A slight or widespread rash may occur.
- Scratching may cause bleeding and skin sores.

#### IMPORTANT POINTS

**Ask for help if:**

- *itching does not disappear after two days.*
- *the person's skin takes on a yellowish colour.*
- *the person scratches so much that the skin is raw.*
- *the rash becomes worse after creams or ointments have been applied.*

### How you can offer care

Scratching without thinking or during sleep may be difficult to control. The main comfort you can provide is finding ways to soothe the itching skin.

- Apply skin creams with a water-soluble base two to three times a day, especially after a bath when the skin is damp.
- Use warm water instead of hot for bathing, as hot water dries the skin.
- Add baking soda or bath oil to the bath water.
- Wash skin gently using a mild soap. Do not scrub.
- Use baking soda instead of deodorant under the arms.
- Keep nails clean and short.
- Encourage the use of rubbing, pressure or vibration instead of scratching.
- Choose loose clothing made of a soft fabric.
- Change bed sheets daily.
- If the person's condition can tolerate it, help keep body fluid levels up by encouraging the person to drink water and other liquids.
- Provide diversions such as television, radio, and books.
- Cover the person with lightweight bedding.
- Avoid scented and alcohol-based products on the skin.
- Use gentle laundry detergents.

## IMPORTANT POINTS

*An open sore on the skin surface or underlying tissue needs urgent attention.*

*Ask for help if:*

- *you notice cracked, blistered, scaly, broken or reddened skin.*
- *the sore is getting larger.*
- *the sore smells foul.*
- *you notice thick green liquid draining from the sore.*

## BED SORES (PRESSURE SORES)

A bed sore develops when the oxygen flow to a particular area of the body is stopped and the tissue in that area dies. The sores are made worse when the person rubs against the sheets, is pulled up against the bed sheets or chair fabric causing friction, or is left with urine or a bowel movement on the skin for too long.

### What you need to know

The best approach to bed sores is prevention. (see Attention to Skin Pressure Areas, page 36). They are very difficult to heal in the seriously ill once they occur. The first hint of a sore is a sign for extra care.

- Red areas on the skin that do not go away, even if the pressure is removed, are a warning that a sore may develop.
- Cracked, blistered, scaly, or broken skin can break down very easily.
- Pain at the "pressure points" (back of head, back of shoulders, elbows, buttocks, and heels) are a warning that these areas need special attention. (See Figure 26.)
- Yellowish-colored stains on clothing, sheets or chair (that may also be tinged with blood) are probably from an oozing sore.

### How you can offer care

Being bedridden, or always in a wheelchair, puts constant pressure on the same places. This makes such areas more likely to develop sores. If sores appear, keep them clean and allow no further pressure on the area. Tell your home care nurse right away if you find a sore.

- Protect pressure points with pillows to help prevent sores. Check with your home care nurse for items that may be suggested to help, such as heel pads and elbow pads.
- Ask your home care nurse about the possibility of changing to a mattress that reduces pressure.
- Have the person move and sit in a chair every day if possible.

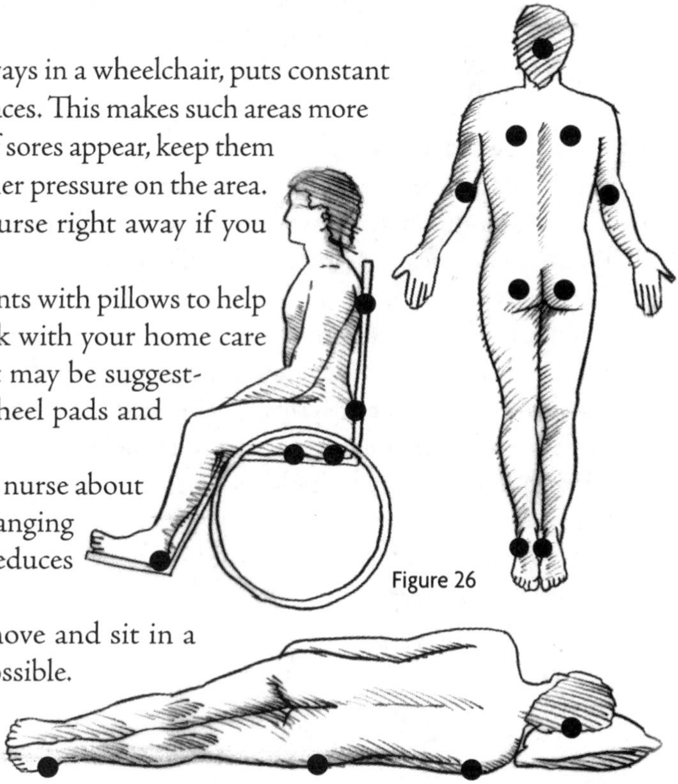

Figure 26

- Lift, rather than pull, the person when changing positions.
- Keep sheets pulled tight to prevent wrinkles.
- Keep the head of the bed flat or up at a 30-degree angle so there is less pressure at the base of the spine.
- Depending on the condition and disease progression, aim to move the person in bed every two hours from left side, to back, to right side. This turning could be continued every four hours through the night.
- Change the bed immediately and clean the skin if the person has urine or a bowel movement on the skin.
- When the person is eating well, encourage them to eat high protein foods.

# MOUTH PROBLEMS

■

## THRUSH (ORAL CANDIDIASIS)

Thrush occurs commonly in people with advanced illness. It is most likely to occur after the person has been on steroids or antibiotics, and is common after radiation of the mouth.

### What you need to know

A thrush infection needs careful attention.

- Your loved one may complain of a sore mouth, sore throat, dry scratchy throat, hoarseness, or problems swallowing.
- When you inspect the mouth, you may see white curd-like patches on the tongue, roof of the mouth, inside the cheeks and lips, and back of the throat.
- Thrush is treated with the medication nystatin (such as Mycostatin™, Nadostine™, Nilstat™, or Nystex™). The medication is a liquid that is swished in the mouth like a mouthwash, then swallowed.
- The doctor may prescribe a medicated cream to rub on the gums under dentures.
- Thrush can spread to others. Avoid kissing the person on the lips or sharing utensils if you suspect thrush.

### How you can offer care

Before each dose of medication is taken, the mouth should be well cleaned. (See the section *Mouth Care*, page 33 for guidance on doing this.)

- Tell your home care nurse immediately if you suspect thrush.
- Use a new toothbrush before treatment begins and replace it again when all the medication is finished.
- Help the person rinse well with clear water before taking the medication.
- Remove dentures before medication is taken.
- Clean dentures well at each treatment. If they are not cleaned properly, they can re-infect the mouth.
- Soak the dentures each night in a solution of one part vinegar to four parts water.

## MOUTH SORES

Mouth sores are like little cuts or ulcers in the mouth. Chemotherapy, radiation therapy, infection, limited fluid intake, poor mouth care, oxygen therapy, too much alcohol or tobacco use, and some medications can cause them.

### What you need to know

Mouth sores can be very painful and interfere with eating and drinking.

- Small ulcers or sores in mouth, on gums, or on the tongue may be seen.
- The sores may be red, bleed or have small white patches in the middle.
- The inside of the mouth, gums and tongue may look red, shiny or swollen.
- There may be blood or pus in the mouth.
- A white or yellow film in the mouth may occur.
- Food that is eaten may cause dryness or mild burning.
- There may be sensitivity to hot and cold.
- Increased or decreased mucus in the mouth may be a problem.
- The person may have difficulty swallowing.
- A sore throat or a burning sensation in the upper chest may be a symptom.
- Check with your home care nurse and doctor for help.

### How you can offer care

- Offer mouth care to help ease the discomfort, with soothing products and non-irritating food and drink.
- Check the mouth twice a day using a small flashlight and tongue blade. If the person wears dentures, remove these first.
- Tell your home care nurse if the person's mouth looks different or there is a change in taste or sensation.
- Do mouth care 30 minutes after eating and every two hours while the person is awake and their condition can tolerate it.
- Use one of the suggested rinsing solutions after mouth care (see *Dry Mouth*, below).
- Apply a water-soluble lubricant such as Muco™ or K-Y Jelly™ to help soothe the lips.
- When possible, encourage the person to drink more fluids if they can be tolerated at this stage of illness.
- Offer small, frequent, cold, non-spicy, bland meals as the person tolerates.
- Try chilled foods and fluids (popsicles, ice cubes, frozen yogurt, sherbet, or ice cream).
- Avoid citrus fruits and juices such as oranges, lemons, limes, and tomatoes. Although they may seem to moisten the mouth, they actually have a drying effect.

## DRY MOUTH

Dry mouth may occur when a person's advanced condition means they are not able to drink and/or absorb the usual volume of liquids. This may happen with nausea, vomiting, or a lack of appetite due to symptoms and advanced illness. The reduced fluid will cause saliva to dry up. Some medications and mouth breathing can also cause dry mouth.

### What you need to know

Dry mouth can be a source of discomfort for a person.

- The complaint may be a dry mouth or a bad taste in the mouth.
- The person's tongue may be red and coated, and the lips dry and cracked.

### How you can offer care

The most helpful thing you can do is keep your loved one's mouth clean and moist, to help it feel fresh.

- Help the person to clean the mouth often, especially after eating and before bed (see Mouth Care, page 33). A rinsing solution suggested by your home care nurse or doctor may help moisten the mouth.
- Put a water-soluble lubricant such as Muco™ or K-Y Jelly™ on the lips after cleaning.
- Try to keep a bowl of ice chips by the bed. Even if the person does not want or is unable to drink, suggest sucking ice cubes to moisten the mouth.
- Try a commercial moistening product recommended by your home care nurse, doctor or pharmacist.
- Remove dentures, rub a moistening product over the gums, then replace the dentures or keep them out, depending on the person's preference.
- Do not use commercial mouthwashes.

## IMPORTANT POINTS

- *Always use an ultra-soft toothbrush. A hard brush can damage fragile gum tissue.*
- *Avoid commercial mouthwashes that contain alcohol. These can all cause more drying and pain.*
- *Do not use dental floss as it can damage gum tissue.*
- *Encourage the person to avoid tobacco or alcohol. These can aggravate mouth sores.*
- *If mouth sores are severe, leave dentures out except for eating.*
- *Avoid hard and coarse foods such as crackers, raw vegetables, and potato chips.*

**Ask for help if:**

- *the thrush or sores do not improve.*
- *drinking and swallowing are affected.*
- *redness and shininess appear in the mouth.*
- *a dry mouth lasts for more than 48 hours.*
- *temperature goes above normal.*

# BOWEL AND BLADDER PROBLEMS

■

## INCONTINENCE

Incontinence is lack of control of the bowels or bladder.

### What you need to know

- For some people, the best choice for controlling regular ongoing incontinence of urine is use of a catheter.
- A catheter is a tube put in the bladder so the urine can drain into a specially designed bag.

### How you can offer comfort and care

- Skin breakdown, which can be caused by pressure and contact with urine or a bowel movement, is a risk from incontinence. Clean and dry skin is very important in preventing this skin breakdown.
- Consider special incontinence garments (e.g. Stayfree™, DryPlus™, Attends™, Poise™, Ensure Guards™) which are available at drugstores and supermarkets. They keep the bed dry and should be changed often. Your home care nurse can give you advice about these. You may be able to get financial assistance to cover their cost (see Appendix I Financial Aid, page 146).
- Use water-repellent creams containing zinc oxide and silicone (e.g. Zincofax™, Penaten Cream™, A&D Cream™) applied as needed to help prevent skin irritation. A silicone and zinc oxide spray (e.g. Silon™) may be available and may be easier to use.
- When the person has a permanent catheter, wash the area where the catheter enters the body at least once a day with soap and water to protect the skin and prevent infection.
- Wash your hands before and after touching the catheter, drainage bag or incontinence garments.
- Check the drainage tubing for kinks and make sure the drainage bag is below the level of the person to encourage draining by gravity.
- Empty the drainage bag at least twice a day.

## IMPORTANT POINTS

*Ask for help if:*

- *there is leaking around where the catheter enters the body.*
- *the urine becomes cloudy, has an offensive smell, or the person develops a sudden fever. These could indicate a bladder infection.*
- *there is blood in the urine.*
- *the person is having diarrhea.*

## CONSTIPATION

When a person has a bowel movement, stool (feces) is passed. Constipation means infrequency or difficulty passing stool. Due to the progressive illness constipation can happen because of:

- medications such as opioids.
- less drinking.
- less eating.
- low fibre in diet.
- less physical activity.
- the type of progressive illness.

Constipation must be assessed and verified by your home care nurse and doctor to make sure there is not an obstruction that may also be interfering with the passing of stool.

### What you need to know

- Stool is still produced even when the person is not eating.
- Constipation is uncomfortable and may cause serious problems. Keeping ahead of it through prevention is very important.
- Stool may be dry and painful to pass.
- The person may have large amounts of gas, burping, or feel sick to the stomach.
- There may be pain in the abdomen.
- What may appear to be diarrhea may in fact be small amounts of runny stool escaping around the hard constipated stool.
- The person may have small hard bowel movements, but not enough stool to correct the constipation.
- Headaches and possibly confusion may accompany constipation.
- The person's abdomen may look blown-up or bloated.

- The doctor may prescribe a stimulant and or laxative medication that can come in the form of a pill, liquid or a suppository (see Giving Medications by Suppository, page 64).
- Some people with constipation are not able to take or do not respond to medications or diet changes and may need an enema.

## IMPORTANT POINTS

- *Keep a daily diary of the person's bowel movements. Even if someone has not been eating or drinking much, contact your home care nurse if a bowel movement has not occurred in two days.*
- *Avoid bulk laxatives such as Metamucil™. A person must drink three litres of fluid a day for these to be effective. Otherwise, they just make the problem worse.*

**Ask for help if:**

- *there is blood in or around anal area or in stool.*
- *there is no bowel movement within one day after taking a laxative.*
- *the person has persistent cramps or vomiting.*

### How you can offer comfort and care

If you are aware of the causes, you may be able to take steps to prevent constipation. Keeping the stage of the advanced illness in mind, consider whether the following strategies might be tolerated:

- Try gradually increasing the intake of fiber and whole grains in cereals and breads. At the same time, a large amount of fluid must be taken in to move the fibre through the system.
- Increase fluid intake.
- Offer a hot drink with caffeine in the morning to encourage a bowel movement.
- Encourage the person to walk, exercise or move about in bed.
- Avoid foods that can cause constipation such as chocolate, cheese and eggs.
- Remind the person of the need to take prescribed laxatives especially if opioids are being used (see Possible Side Effects or Complications of Opioids, page 75).
- Offer a variety of fruits (including prunes), vegetables and fruit juices (including prune juice) once a day. The following fruit laxative may be a way to encourage the person to take a variety of these helpful foods.

**FRUIT LAXATIVE** *(use dried fruit)*
- ¼ cup currants • ¼ cup dates
- ¼ cup raisins • ¼ cup figs
- ¼ cup prunes • prune juice

### Bowel routine

Anyone using regular opioids for pain should also use a laxative. A daily basic bowel routine is also advised for someone using opioids. The following is one suggested routine:
- Bowel stimulants and laxatives (e.g. Senokot™ or Lactulose) can be taken once or twice a day.
- Laxatives stimulate increased bowel activity and help to create a bowel movement.
- They can be purchased at the drugstore and their cost may be covered by a drug program (see Appendix I *Financial Aid*, page 146).

### Enemas

An enema is fluid injected into the rectum to clean out the bowel. To give a small enema such as a Fleet™, the same procedure is followed as for suppositories.
- Help the person into a position that will make it easy to insert the enema tube. The best position is lying on the left side, with the upper leg bent forward. (There should be a diagram on the instructions that come with the enema.)
- Advise the person that the enema may cause a feeling of pressure and cramps. Encourage them to take deep breaths and hold the enema in as long as possible before expelling.
- The tube will already be lubricated.
- Insert the tube gently into the rectum and squeeze the container.
- Go slowly but try not to stop if the person has discomfort. Use the full enema or as much as the person can tolerate.

## DIARRHEA

Diarrhea is the passage of loose or watery bowel movements three or more times a day. There may or may not be discomfort. Causes of diarrhea include infections, some medications, surgery, fistulas, laxatives, side effects of chemotherapy, radiation therapy to the abdomen, and sometimes the disease itself.

### What you need to know

- Diarrhea can upset the body's balance of salts and chemicals called electrolytes.
- Certain foods can make diarrhea worse while other foods may help slow it.
- Dehydration is always a risk from severe diarrhea.
- Diarrhea can also be the overflow of liquid stool around hard stool. In this case, it should be treated as constipation (see Constipation, page 87). Ask your home care nurse about this possibility.

### IMPORTANT POINTS

- *Avoid foods that may stimulate or irritate the digestive tract. Examples are whole grain bread and cereal, fried or greasy food, nuts, raw fruits or vegetables, rich pastries, strong spices and herbs, caffeinated foods or drinks, alcoholic or carbonated beverages, and tobacco products.*
- *Very hot or very cold foods can trigger diarrhea.*
- *Avoid giving only clear liquids for more than two days in a row.*

**Ask for help if:**

- *the person has six or more loose bowel movements more than two days in a row.*
- *you notice blood in or around the anal area or in the bowel movement.*

### How you can offer comfort and care

If possible, food and fluid should be the choice for restoring the fluid balance of the body.

- Choose foods high in protein, calories and potassium. Talk to your dietitian or home care nurse about suitable foods.
- If the person can drink more fluids, aim for eight to 10 glasses of fluid daily. Sipping slowly helps fluids absorb better.
- Make sure water is not the only fluid taken. Serve a variety of drinks and jelly products such as Jello™.
- Try frequent small meals instead of three large meals.
- Wash the anal area with mild soap and pat dry after each bowel movement.
- Apply a water-repellent product (Zincofax™, Penaten Cream™, A&D Cream™, Silon™) to the anal area to protect the skin.
- Be calm when diarrhea occurs. Try to reduce the person's anxiety and embarrassment with the situation.
- Use protective pads on the bed to lessen embarrassment and help with clean-up.
- Use a room deodorizer if odour is a problem.

# SHORTNESS OF BREATH (DYSPNEA)

■

Shortness of breath, also called dyspnea, occurs when the body cannot get enough oxygen. Either the lungs cannot take in enough air, or they cannot deliver enough oxygen to the blood stream. Shortness of breath has many causes, including illness, anxiety or pollution (including tobacco smoke).

## What you need to know

Severe shortness of breath can be frightening for both the person experiencing it and anyone watching. Knowing what to expect may make it less disturbing.

- The skin around the mouth and nail beds may become blue-tinged.
- There may be large amounts of thick mucus that the person can or cannot cough up.
- Respirations may sound moist and gurgling.
- Breathing may be difficult when moving, talking, or even resting.
- Depending on the cause of the shortness of breath and the stage of the progressive illness, some treatment may be considered. Medication and other interventions may also be offered.

## How you can offer comfort and care

- Your loved one may have less trouble breathing if the surroundings are calm and you follow certain guidelines.
- Encourage the quiet presence of a calm supportive family member or friend to help ease the anxiety.
- Plan frequent rest periods between activities if the shortness of breath is worse with movement, washing, dressing or talking.
- Ask visitors just to sit quietly and calmly so there is no need to talk.
- Be sure medication and other interventions prescribed for shortness of breath is taken as directed.
- Use a humidifier may help loosen mucus, making it easier for the person coughing.
- Avoid standing over or too close to the person. Open a window or use a fan to help give a sense of more surrounding air.
- Remove tight or constricted clothing. Use a lightweight blanket as bedding.
- Remember to remain calm in the person's presence. Your distress can make your loved one more anxious, increasing the breathlessness.

- Help the person to a position that makes breathing easier. Lying flat often makes shortness of breath worse. Usually a high sitting position is best. Put several pillows or a special seat support pillow at the back. Another helpful position involves leaning on a bed table or high table with the head resting on crossed arms.
- Try a recliner chair for sleep as it keeps the body in a semi-upright position.
- Do whatever you can to help the person remain relaxed, as tense muscles add to breathlessness.
- Medications such as opioids may be prescribed to relieve shortness of breath.

## IMPORTANT POINTS

**Ask for help if:**

- *the person complains of chest pain.*
- *thick, yellow, green or bloody mucus is being produced.*
- *the person cannot get a proper breath for three minutes.*
- *the skin is pale or blue or the person feels cold and clammy.*
- *there is a fever.*
- *the nostrils flare during breathing.*

## OXYGEN THERAPY

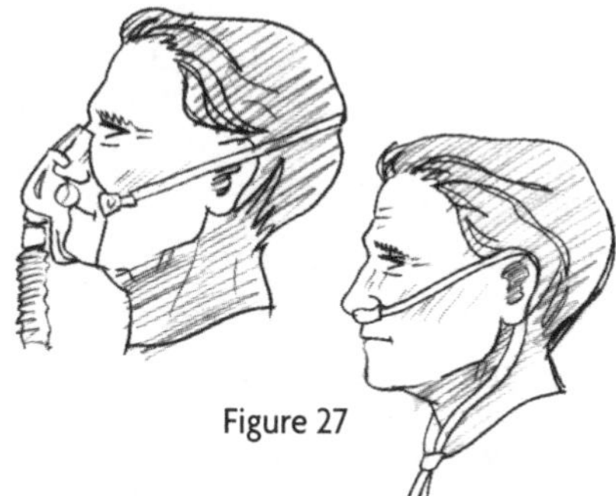
Figure 27

### What you need to know

Sometimes the doctor will recommend oxygen therapy to help ease shortness of breath. Oxygen can be given in two ways:

- through a nose cannula – a short, plastic, disposable tubing that enters the person's nostrils. (See Figure 27.)
- or using a disposable plastic face mask. It fits over the nose and mouth firmly and is attached to the oxygen supply.

### How you can offer comfort and care

A mask or cannula needs attention to be as comfortable as possible.

- Remove and clean the mask as needed.
- Place something soft such as small cotton pads or moleskin between the tubing and the skin to lessen irritation.
- Tighten the elastic on a mask so that it fits snugly on the person's face.
- The prongs of the nasal cannula must be in the person's nose.
- Oxygen can dry the inside of the nose. A water-based, non-prescription preparation, such as Secaris™, can help.

### IMPORTANT POINTS

- *Oxygen can fuel a fire.*
- *Do not smoke or light matches in a room where oxygen is in use.*
- *Do not use oxygen around a gas stove.*
- *Do not use oil-based products such as Vaseline™ or mineral oil close to oxygen.*
- *Use oxygen only as the doctor directs. This may be 24 hours a day or only part of the time.*
- *Oxygen is needed most during activity, such as getting in and out of bed, a chair or the tub, on outings, and when walking.*
- *Make sure a 24 hour supply of oxygen is available, especially on weekends and holidays.*
- *Follow the supplier's instructions to ensure that the equipment works properly.*
- *Know the number of the supplier to call if you have a problem.*
- *In order to use oxygen at home, you may need a house inspection and approval from your fire department.*

# NAUSEA AND VOMITING

■

Nausea means feeling sick to the stomach and vomiting means throwing up. Nausea can happen even when a person is not thinking about food. Vomiting can occur even if nothing has been eaten or there has been no nausea.

Many things can cause nausea and vomiting. These can include the illness, medications, irritation of the digestive system, certain foods, constipation, pain, bowel obstruction, infection, anxiety, movement, and some treatments. Sometimes the cause has nothing to do with the illness, and is as simple as having the flu.

**What you need to know**

Everyone experiences nausea and vomiting at some point. For a person with an advanced illness, the difference may be the frequency and intensity, made worse by the weakness that accompanies the illness.

- The person may feel sick and unable to eat.
- Vomiting may happen occasionally or often.
- Medications taken by mouth may be vomited.
- The person may be comfortable at rest but feel sick with movement.

**How you can offer comfort and care**

The comfort you can offer is aimed mostly at reducing any triggers that might cause nausea and/or vomiting, and providing doctor-ordered medications by different routes to try to ease or relieve it. If and when it does ease:

- Try offering small amounts of favorite foods and fluids as tolerated.
- Try cold foods because they have less odour.
- Keep a supply of clear fluids, ice chips, frozen juice chips, and ginger ale to offer in small quantities.
- Cooking smells may stimulate nausea. Try to keep these away from the sick person.
- Do not offer greasy or spicy foods. Try bland foods such as crackers, toast, angel food cake, soft fruits and yogurt.
- Encourage the person to take the anti-nausea medication regularly, as directed by the home care nurse or doctor.
- Freshen the mouth with a non-alcohol based mouthwash or club soda.
- Always keep clean basins close by. If vomiting occurs, replace the basin right away.

- Open windows or use a fan to see if air helps to reduce the sensation of nausea.
- Help the person to rest sitting up for an hour to aid digestion after meals.
- Encourage anyone who will be close to the person to avoid using perfumes, aftershaves or deodorants with strong fragrances.
- Ask your doctor, home care nurse or pharmacist if complementary care suggestions such as herbal remedies might help (see Herbal Remedies, page 108).

## IMPORTANT POINTS

- *If vomiting occurs in bed, position the person on one side so that vomit will not be inhaled and cause choking.*
- *Keep a record of how often and how much the person vomits.*
- *Depending on the cause of the nausea or vomiting, the doctor will order appropriate medications or interventions to try.*

*Ask for help if:*

- *vomiting occurs more than three times an hour for three or more hours.*
- *blood or material that looks like coffee grounds appears in the vomit.*
- *the person has been eating and drinking well, but nausea and vomiting no longer allows it.*
- *medications are vomited.*
- *the person now feels unusually weak and dizzy.*
- *the person suddenly becomes unresponsive.*

# TROUBLE SLEEPING (INSOMNIA)

■

Insomnia means the inability to sleep properly when sleep would normally be expected. It may range from disturbed sleep to being fully awake.

### What you may expect

At one time or another, most people who are seriously ill have difficulty falling asleep or staying asleep.

- Insomnia may be caused by anxiety, fear, sadness or other psychological or spiritual concerns.
- Physical problems such as pain, nausea, vomiting and coughing may cause insomnia.

## IMPORTANT POINTS

*Do not ignore symptoms such as pain, nausea, or coughing that may lead to insomnia. Give medications that have been prescribed.*

**Ask for help if:**

- *the person becomes confused at night time.*
- *you are not sleeping and need relief.*

### How you can offer comfort and care

A person who has a serious illness may sleep a lot during the day. When the usual time to sleep arrives at night, insomnia may be present.

- Allow the person to sleep whenever, and as much as needed, without staying to a schedule.
- Provide warm, non-caffeinated drinks such as warm milk with honey before sleep.
- Spend quiet times with the person, listening and talking. The opportunity to express feelings will do much to relieve a person's emotional concerns.
- Try to make the person comfortable. Close contact such as holding a hand, sitting or lying nearby on the bed may give comfort.
- Offer backrubs or massage the feet to help with relaxation.
- Keep sheets clean and as free from wrinkles as possible.
- Be sure the area is quiet when the person wants to sleep.
- Ask your home care nurse or doctor if any medications or other therapies could help.

# SWELLING (EDEMA)

■

Edema is common in people with advanced cancer and end stage heart, lung, liver and renal diseases. Edema occurs when tiny blood vessels in your body (capillaries) leak fluid. The fluid builds up in surrounding tissues, leading to swelling in parts of the body such as the legs and abdomen. Edema can also occur if a progressive illness makes protein hard to replace in the body, or if there are tumours or obstructions to the veins or lymph system. Unless the swelling is related to a heart problem, water pills will not be effective in removing extra fluid. Your doctor or home care nurse can explain why your loved one is experiencing edema.

### What you may expect

When fluid accumulates, some easily identified changes take place:

- The feet and lower legs swell when the person sits, stands or walks.
- Rings become too tight for the fingers.
- The person complains of 'tightness' in the hands when making a fist.
- The abdomen looks distended or blown up, or the person complains of tight pants or shortness of breath.

### How you can offer comfort and care

In an advanced illness, the most that you as caregiver can do to address and provide comfort for the edema is:

- Encourage bed rest.
- If feet are swollen, elevate feet. When the person is seated, keep the feet elevated on a stool with a pillow,
- If the arms are swollen, rest them on a table, cushioned on a pillow, to elevate them.
- Ask if any exercises may be helpful.
- Massage swollen areas to help fluid absorb.
- Use compression stockings or bandages when the person is sitting.

## IMPORTANT POINTS

**Ask for help if:**

- *you press your finger into the swollen area and the finger mark stays.*
- *swelling spreads up legs or arms.*
- *swelling in the belly causes shortness of breath.*

# LOSS OF STRENGTH

■

Loss of strength may be a result of the advancing progressive illness or come from weakened muscles after a prolonged stay in bed. It usually occurs gradually, but can sometimes happen over just a few days.

## What you may expect

A person who was once active and independent will usually have difficulty adjusting to the physical limitations of a progressive illness. If you understand how weakness affects the body, you can plan your care accordingly.

- Tiredness is common after activities that once were easy.
- The person may need help to walk, bath or dress, or may need to be cared for in bed.
- It may be difficult for the person to move in bed and get from one place to another.
- Frustration with physical limitations may make the person irritable during situations that would normally pass unnoticed.

## How you can offer comfort and care

Your care will focus on helping your loved one save and space out energy during activities.

- Ask a member of the health care team to teach you techniques for helping a person move more easily while conserving energy.
- Reassure the person that you wish to help. Someone who is losing strength often becomes upset about being dependent.
- Put a bell, a spoon and tin plate, or anything that can be used to make a noise to call you when needed. Baby monitors also work well.
- Remind the person about the need to limit activities and to rest before doing any activity.
- Ask a member of your health care team if a walker, wheelchair or other aids would help. You may be able to buy or rent equipment. (see Appendix VI *Further Medical, Legal and Financial Provincial Contacts*, page 154).

# CONFUSION

■

A person who has trouble thinking and acting appropriately or has disturbed thoughts is said to be confused. A person with a progressive illness may become confused due to the illness, infection, a side effect of medications, decreased fluids, or during the final days. Tell your home care nurse if you notice the start of confusion and ask if anything can be tried to help.

## What you need to know

At some point, confusion often goes hand-in-hand with a progressive physical illness. Understanding how a confused person might act may help you to feel less anxious when you see unfamiliar behaviours.

- Confusion can start very slowly.
- It can appear as poor concentration, loss of memory and of interest.
- Making decisions may be difficult because of poor concentration.
- The person may describe a sense of unreality or the feeling of "losing my mind."
- Feelings may fluctuate between denial and acceptance of the situation.
- A confused person may become restless and move about in a random fashion. There may appear to be pain.
- The person may hallucinate (see or hear things that are not real), particularly at night.
- Strange thoughts may bother the person.
- Fear and anger may appear for no obvious reason.
- Movements may become slow or agitated.
- Confusion can become so severe that the person cannot make proper decisions. In this case, having an advanced care plan and substitute decision maker in place will help in making health decisions and taking legal responsibility for affairs.

### How you can offer comfort and care

Since harm can come easily to a confused person, close supervision and guidance are needed.

- When appropriate, quietly remind the person who you are whenever it seems necessary.
- If it does not cause agitation, gently touch the person during conversations to remind that you are there.
- Stand face to face and stay within a respectful space of the person when talking.
- Turn off radio and TV, and do not play them together or loudly.
- Talk slowly and quietly, using short statements.
- Aim to be a quiet presence that supports the confused person. Be aware that trying to correct the confusion or hallucinations may cause more agitation.
- Consider keeping a calendar and clock in view. When asked, you can try to gently remind them of what day and time it is.
- Keep the room well-lit, unless light is disturbing.
- Do not give medications or any care without explaining what you are doing.
- Do not leave the person alone.
- Use preventative measures to reduce the chance of the person falling out of a chair or bed.

## IMPORTANT POINTS

**Ask for help if:**

- *confusion occurs very suddenly or becomes worse.*
- *the person becomes violent or very agitated.*
- *you or the person is hurt because of the confusion.*
- *you are tired and need relief.*

# COMPLEMENTARY CARE

■

The word complementary suggests care techniques that are used along with conventional medicine. You might consider using the following techniques in your home to help your loved one feel more comfortable. They are not intended as a substitute for medical care. Never use them without checking first with a member of your health care team. You may want to explore other available types of complementary care. Discuss these ideas with your home care nurse or doctor.

## RELAXATION TECHNIQUES

Since the main purpose of using relaxation aids is to focus your loved one on an activity and away from the discomfort of illness, anything you can do to provide distraction is helpful. Never use relaxation techniques as a substitute for pain relief medications.

### How you can offer comfort

Techniques for relaxation involve a conscious attempt to relax all the muscles. These are more structured than we usually mean when we think of relaxing. All relaxation techniques begin in the same way.

- Choose a quiet room.
- Try to avoid interruptions during the time of the chosen activity. Hang a 'Do Not Disturb' sign on the door if needed.
- Choose a time that feels right, such as:
  - before pain or discomfort is severe.
  - when the person feels worried or nervous.
  - at the same time every day.
- Ask if any favorite music would offer added relaxation.
- Help the person settle into a comfortable position, with the arms and legs relaxed.
- Begin the activity by having the person breathe in deeply through the nose and out slowly through the mouth, as though whistling. Do this three times. (Do not encourage a person with breathing problems to do deep breathing exercises.)
- Encourage the person to keep the eyes closed and focus on how the activity feels.
- Have the person think of a calm, peaceful place and picture being very light, floating, or nice and warm.
- After the activity, ask for feedback so you know what worked and what did not.

## IMAGERY

Imagery relaxation uses the imagination to help someone relax. It is a way to 'picture' something to take the mind off discomfort.

### What you do

- Remind the person of the previous preparation for relaxation techniques.
- Provide ideas for images of pain relief. For example:
  - imagine the pain as a large rock that is part of the body. Next, visualize a large helium balloon tied to the rock, lifting the rock and the pain away.
  - feel pain as a thunderstorm that rains on the body, then imagine that a gentle breeze blows the thunderstorm and the pain away.
  - remember a special place where the person has been that creates its own pain-easing images.
- Help the person do the imagery relaxation 20 minutes a day.

## RELAXATION BREATHING

Relaxation breathing is a technique of breathing in a controlled way to relax tense muscles and take the mind off discomfort.

### What you need

- Music player (with or without headphones).
- Relaxation tapes/music to help the person work through the relaxation breathing.

### What you do

- Remind the person of the preparation for relaxation techniques.
- Make the relaxation tape the focus of the exercise.
- Breathing exercises are done in a rotation.
- Breathe in deeply through the nose. At the same time, tense a muscle or group of muscles – make a fist or clench the teeth.
- Hold the breath and tense muscles for one to two seconds.
- Relax the muscles and breathe out slowly.
- Tense the muscles in the lower right leg while breathing in deeply.
- Relax the muscles in the lower right leg while breathing out slowly.
- Repeat with the lower left leg, then slowly work all the way up the body. Each time, tense the muscles while breathing in deeply and relax while breathing out slowly.
- Encourage using these exercises for at least 20 minutes a day.
- Avoid relaxation tapes that may cause bad or worrying thoughts or physical pain.

- With someone who has problems breathing, focus on just relaxing for a minute or two before starting the exercises instead of doing deep breathing.

## VIBRATION MASSAGE

Vibration massage is a massage using an electric device. It helps to numb the area of pain and to relax tense muscles.

### What you need

- Electric massager

### What you do

- Choose the area of the body where there is pain.
- Remove clothing from the area.
- Cover areas not being massaged, for warmth and privacy.
- Find positions in which you will both be comfortable.
- Massage an area below or above the pain if the actual area is too painful to touch.
- Rather than massaging the area of pain directly, try using the massager on the opposite side of the body. For instance, if the right hip hurts, try the massager on the left hip.
- Do not do vigorous massage over the area of a tumour.
- Apply the massager for 25 to 45 minutes, twice a day.
- Turn the massager on and off every few seconds for 25 to 45 minutes if that is more comfortable.
- Follow the instructions on the electric massager to avoid electrical shock.

## DISTRACTION

Any technique that helps distract a person from immediate discomfort can be helpful. Begin by preparing the area as you would for relaxation techniques.

### Music

Music has the power to absorb some people so totally that they forget everything else for a while. Using headphones to block out other sounds, can make the distraction even more complete.

### What you need

- Radio, CD, cassette player, iPod or the latest music player (with or without headphones) with the music the person likes.

### What you do

- Help the person choose some favourite music.

- Encourage singing along with the music, or keeping time by tapping with fingers and feet to the beat.
- Try using music distraction several times a day.

### Humour

Laughter can lift a person's mood and even ease pain. Distracting with humour helps your loved one focus on something other than the discomfort.

#### What you need

- Comedy audio or video tapes and players, television, radio

#### What you can do

- Find out what type of humour the person is in the mood to enjoy - maybe British comedy or slapstick.
- Help with the choice of a comedy audio or videotape.
- Share jokes, funny cartoons and stories.

## COMFORT FROM COLD TREATMENTS

Applying cold to the body has many benefits. It reduces muscles spasms, numbs nerve endings, reduces swelling and eases itching.

- Cold that is to be left in one place, rather than massaged over an area, should be wrapped in a cloth.
- Leave the cold on for at least 10 to 15 minutes. It can be left on for up to 30 minutes.
- Do this three to four times a day.
- Switch back and forth from cold to heat if that provides comfort.
- Try applying heat rubs and ointments such as Ben Gay™, Rub A.535™, Tiger Balm™ to the painful area before using the ice cold treatment.
- Do not use a cold rub cream such as Icy Cold™ at the same time as any other cold treatment.
- Test creams or ointments on the inside of an arm first to be sure they do not irritate the skin. If there is no redness or itching after a few minutes, try it on the area of pain.
- Wash your hands after putting on creams. Be sure you do not get any cream near your eyes.

### Ice bags

These bags are used to apply cold to a painful area.

### What you need

An ice bag made up from one of the following:

- commercial ice bag.
- Ziploc™ bag filled with crushed or shaved ice.
- bag containing small pieces of frozen food such as corn, peas or unpopped popcorn kernels.
- towel or pillowcase.
- heat rub (optional).

### What you do

- If using a Ziploc™ bag filled with ice, push all of the air out of the bag.
- Hit a bag of frozen vegetables on the counter top to break them up.
- Place the ice bag in a pillowcase or towel. If the person wants it colder, wet the covering.
- Place the ice bag on the area with pain. If this causes more pain, put the ice bag above or below the area.
- Refreeze the bag of vegetables after use, making sure to mark the bag so you do not eat the product.

## Cold cloths

Cold cloths are simply applied to a painful area.

### What you need

- Two towels
- Ice
- Basin
- Heat rub (optional)

#### What you do

- Fill the basin with two inches of water.
- Add ice to the water.
- Soak the towels in the ice water.
- Wring out a towel and place it on the area that hurts.
- When the towel becomes warm, put it back in the ice water and repeat with the second towel.

### Cold or ice massage

This involves massaging ice or cold onto a painful area.

#### What you need

- Ice
- Towel and wash cloth
- Plastic bag or garbage bag
- Paper cup

#### What you do

- Fill a paper cup halfway with water.
- Put the cup in the freezer until the water is frozen solid.
- Peel the cup to uncover the ice.
- Cover the plastic bag with the towel. Place it under the area that will be massaged to catch water as it melts.
- Wrap a wash cloth around the paper cup to stop your hands from getting cold.
- Rub the ice in a circle over the area that hurts.
- Dry the skin with the towel as the ice melts.
- Massage the area for about four minutes. It is normal for the area to get red.

## COMFORT FROM HEAT TREATMENTS

Heat can be soothing and also has beneficial effects by relaxing tense muscles. There are two important things to remember:

- use caution when using electric heating pads, especially those that do not automatically turn off, as they can cause burns.
- do not use heat rubs when using heat treatments.

## Hot water bottles

Most households have a hot water bottle. It can be used with little preparation.

### What you do

- Fill the bottle with water from the hot water tap. Do not use boiling water as it can be difficult to judge how hot the bottle will become.
- After putting in the stopper, shake the bottle gently to be sure it will not leak.
- Cover the bottle with a towel or similar cover so there is no direct contact with skin.
- Prop it against the area where the person is having discomfort.

## Microwave heat bags

These bags can be heated in the microwave and are used to put heat on an area.

### What you need

- Microwave
- Flax seed bag or specially formulated heat pack
- Fleece cover or towel

### How you do it

- Put the bag in the microwave and microwave on high for two minutes.
- Wrap the bag in the fleece cover or towel. Never use a hot pack without a cover.
- Put the bag on the area that hurts.
- If this causes pain, you can put the bag:
  - above or below the area that hurts.
  - on the opposite side of the body. For instance, if the right leg is sore, try the bag on the left leg.
  - Cover the area with blankets to keep the heat in.

## IMPORTANT POINTS

*Be aware of the following when using cold or hot treatments.*

- *Do not use massage, cold or heat on skin that:*
  - *is being radiated.*
  - *has an open wound or sores.*
  - *has bleeding or bruising.*
- *Do not use these treatments if you have been told the person has poor blood flow.*
- *Do not use massage, cold or heat if they increase the pain.*
- *Do not use cold or heat on any area where the person has no sensation (feeling).*

### HERBAL REMEDIES

You and your loved one may be considering a herbal remedy to help with an effect of the terminal illness. Before you do so, remember these important points.

- Herbs have been used for centuries to treat and prevent disease. Some do have healthful properties, but may not be appropriate at the time.
- Many people believe that because herbs are 'natural,' they cannot cause harm. This is simply not true. Herbs are medications in plant form. They have the same potential to cause side effects as other medicines do.
- Herbs can interact with some prescription medications. It is important to tell your home care nurse, doctor or pharmacist if the person you are caring for is using herbal products. Ask about any product if you are uncertain.
- Make sure that any herbs being used are quality products. Most quality products have been tested to ensure they contain a certain percentage of the key ingredient. Also, quality products may have a drug identification number (DIN). The product must have an expiry date and a lot number.
- Avoid any product about which you have doubts.

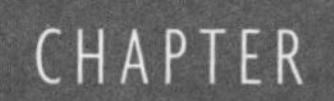

# CHAPTER 4

# AS LIFE ENDS

# PLANNING

■

Planning where the person hopes to spend their final days and receive appropriate end-of-life care is a mutual decision. Communication needs to be open and flexible at all times between the person, the caregivers and health care team. No one can always be completely certain of the type of care that may be needed and is able to be provided as the illness progresses to the final days and hours. By being open and flexible, you will be able to avoid possible future feelings of regret. Remember that the location, especially if it is home, may have to change if symptoms increase, feelings about the location shift, or the caregiver(s) become exhausted and extra support is not available.

Home is often the place that everyone hopes for, since it is familiar and has a lifetime of memories. This may make you feel more in control and closer to family.

Depending on the person's community location, special facilities, units, beds, and teams may also be available to those in the end stage of life. Talk with your home care nurse about what is available and what the access process is in your area.

Plan for what you will do if you or your loved one unable to have, or has a change of mind about, a home death. Remember this is not a failure. You can still ask to help or share guidance with basic care in other settings, ensuring continued connection and comfort.

## DYING AT HOME

What you need to consider:

- The decision to and helping the person die at home can be both rewarding and challenging.
- Talk to your loved one about the arrangements, and mutually share concerns and feelings.
- Learn what you might expect during the last days of your loved one's life. This prepares you for changes you might see and what you can do to provide comfort.
- Tell your home care nurse about religious or other cultural practices that will be important to you and the dying person at that time.

**How you can offer comfort and care:**

Your main role is to offer comfort in any way you can.

- Give recommended interventions and medicine for pain, nausea and shortness of breath and any other symptoms as prescribed.
- Play music or read to your loved one if it seems to be relaxing.
- Reposition your loved one every two hours or a frequently as tolerated, or rearrange the position with pillows.
- Offer back rubs, and maintain skin moisture with lotion.
- Moisten the person's lips, and use lip balm to prevent dryness.
- Be aware of external sounds and determine if these are comforting or upsetting.
- With your loved one's input and direction, monitor and control the number of visitors and the length of the stay so the person does not become exhausted.
- Encourage visitors to phone in advance. Tell them if it is not a good time to come.
- If you have a spiritual leader with a close connection to you and your loved one, keep that person aware of ongoing changes that are happening. Advise if you wish a visit.

## PRACTICAL DETAILS

- Keep the phone numbers of home care nurses, doctors, and other pertinent people accessible and visible - perhaps on the fridge or near your home phone.
- Keep information about care and people to call in a single accessible notebook or on a cell phone.
- Prepare a list of people to call near or at the time of death.
- Decide if a spiritual leader can be called before or at the time of death, if that is what either you or the person wish.
- Ask about the doctor and/or nurse attending at the time of death. Your home care nurse or doctor can explain the process in your community about a pronouncement of an expected home death. This allows you to make prior arrangements.

## IMPORTANT POINTS

- *Prepare for an expected death due to advanced illness that will happen at home. Discussion, clear communications and decisions about allowing the natural process of dying and not trying to revive (resuscitate) the person should take place ahead of time.*
- *Instructions about not performing any resuscitative measures need to be discussed and clearly communicated. This means if an ambulance is needed to transport the person to a hospital, a hospice, or palliative care facility, resuscitation will not be done if the person dies in the ambulance. These instructions are called a Do Not Resuscitate (DNR) order, code status or levels of care. Discuss this with your home care nurse or doctor to make the necessary arrangements.*
- *Tell people who sit with the person or provide nursing care that* **not** *calling 911 is what you and the dying person want and need.*
- *Consider making funeral arrangements ahead of time with a funeral home. Tell them that you are planning a home death. Get information on what you need to do to notify them when death happens.* (see Appendix XI *Canadian Hospice Palliative Care Association*, page 173).
- *If you feel that you are unable to go on caring for the person at home until the end, talk to your loved one, the home care nurse and doctor to consider and plan other arrangements.*

# A MOVE TO HOSPICE, PALLIATIVE CARE, LONG TERM CARE OR HOSPITAL

■

A time may come when your loved one is unable to stay at home. The person may now wish to be admitted to a care facility or hospital, or uncontrolled symptoms related to the advanced illness or difficulty managing care at home may make the move necessary.

### What you need to remember

Being a caregiver is physically and emotionally challenging.

- Do not feel guilty if you find you can no longer provide care at home.
- Continue to stay involved with the person's care, either by helping make decisions or by helping with simple tasks.
- Give yourself permission to take some time away from the person. Consider going back to rest at your home or for a walk. Leave your contact number with the appropriate people.
- Ask family, friends or volunteers to stay with the person if you are uncomfortable leaving your loved one alone.
- Ask the facility about what sleeping, visiting arrangements and support are offered for family if you wish to spend the night.
- Take a book or some activities to do while you sit with your loved one.

## HOW YOU CAN OFFER SUPPORT IF A MOVE FROM HOME IS NEEDED

The decision to move away from the familiar surroundings of home is never easy for anyone. For someone with an advanced terminal illness, the decision may be even more difficult as they are saying a final goodbye to their home.

- Be open, caring and honest with the person about the need to move. Explain the symptoms that need better control or the challenges and limitations you have, and why you are not able to provide the necessary care at home. Enlist the support of your family, friends and care team.
- Involve the person in decisions about anticipated care in the facility to which they will be moving.
- Be with the person during the move.
- Take meaningful objects from home such as family pictures, a quilt, a pillow and clothes to help make the new surroundings more comfortable and familiar.

# LAST DAYS OF LIFE

■

In the final days before death, a person usually goes through changes as the body gradually shuts down.

### What you may expect

## WITHDRAWAL

Someone who is dying may feel a separation from the world. As your loved one is the person going through this, no one else can really understand the total experience. You as the caregiver may feel the person is giving up. Understand and remind yourself that the advanced illness is taking its natural course. The person's condition means they must give in to the normal dying process.

- Many things may happen, such as a life review that examines happy and sad memories, good and strained relationships, losses and thoughts. Beliefs and questions about an after-life may occur as an ongoing process of the advanced illness.
- The person may start to recall or "see" people who have already died.
- The person may be having thoughts that help prepare for and deal with impending death. They may share or not share these with you or others.
- With withdrawal comes less of a need to communicate with others.
- Gentle touch and silence take on more meaning as words lose their importance. This does not mean that the person does not benefit from hearing your words. When you talk with the person, be careful that you are still respectful and caring with your words. Even though there may be no response, it is possible that the person can still hear you.

## CHANGING LEVELS OF AWARENESS

- Advanced illness can affect a person's ability to think clearly and respond to surroundings. Mental changes often coincide with physical changes in the final days of an illness.
- The person may become restless, anxious or irritable for no apparent reason.
- Simple directions may be misunderstood.
- Clear thinking and the ability to communicate thoughts may be diminished.
- Familiar people or objects may not be recognized or simple things forgotten.
- Hallucinations may occur and be troublesome.

- The person may be drowsy all the time and fall asleep even during conversations.
- Sometimes the person may appear to be reaching out, and even call the name of someone who has died.

### How you can offer comfort and care

During the last days of life, the following suggestions may help soothe a person who is withdrawn or distressed.

- Sit quietly as a comforting presence. Use gentle touch as a reminder that you are there or that you want to speak.
- Move close and talk gently. Assume you can be heard even if you do not get a response.
- Reduce confusion by limiting noisy distractions such as television and radio.
- Ask visitors to talk quietly.
- Gently remind the person of the time, who you are and where you both are located.
- If reality is different for the dying person, do not argue about it. Sometimes just listening or agreeing with someone who is mildly confused allows the situation to pass without creating upset.
- Listen quietly if the person needs to express thoughts, worries or feelings.
- Try using soft music for a relaxing effect.
- If the person is alert, swallowing and able to tolerate it, continue to offer drinks and very small portions of favorite foods that are soft and easy to eat.
- Take the food away without a fuss if the person refuses it.
- If tolerated, provide gentle mouth care as a source of comfort at the end of life. Often this is needed, rather than eating or drinking.

# SIGNS THAT DEATH IS APPROACHING

■

### What you need to know

As death is near, the body undergoes changes. If you know what to expect, you will be less anxious and more prepared to see it happening. Remember this is the normal process of dying and that you need not panic or call for medical emergency help or an ambulance. Find out ahead of time if you can connect with your home care nurse or doctor for extra advice, reassurance and support during the final days.

## SIGNS AND SYMPTOMS OF THE DYING PROCESS

- The person has no interest in taking any food or fluids.
- Respirations change, becoming shallow, quicker or slower.
- Breathing may appear difficult, with intermittent periods of no breath.
- Swallowing may become difficult.
- Congestion, bubbling or rattling sounds in the throat and chest may accompany breathing.
- Heartbeat may be irregular.
- Anxiety and restlessness may be present.
- There may be a reduced level of consciousness.
- There is a small quantity of very dark urine or no urine at all.
- There is progressive coldness and purple discoloration, mostly in the arms and legs.
- There may be a loss of bowel and bladder control.

### How you can offer comfort and care

Even if your loved one does not seem to be aware of you during this last stage, your presence is still a comfort.

- Continue to touch, reassuring the person that you are close by and you care.
- Speak calmly and naturally.
- Provide comfort by keeping the person dry and their lips moistened with a lubricant.
- Raise the head of the bed if breathing is difficult, or raise the upper body with pillows.

## IMPORTANT POINTS

- *Your loved one may appear to be in distress with difficult breathing and an irregular heartbeat. However, it may not trouble the person, who may be very comfortable.*
- *Do not try to force liquids or food. This can cause choking and aspiration.*
- *Anything that can be done to ease pain and discomfort, such as medication, massage or gentle touch, is important in these last few hours.*
- *If the person cannot swallow pills, ask the doctor or nurse for advice on alternate routes. It is wise to plan for this possibility ahead of time.*
- *Some of the complementary therapies suggested may be comforting.*
- *Even if your loved one appears to be sleeping or unconscious, your words may be heard and understood. Do not say anything you would not want that person to hear or that might be upsetting.*

# WHEN DEATH OCCURS

■

**What you need to know**

At the time of death, body functions stop.

- There will be no response, no breathing and no pulse.
- The eyes will be fixed in one direction. They may be open or closed.
- The jaws will relax and the mouth may open slightly.
- There may be loss of control of bladder or bowels.

## WHAT TO DO IF DEATH HAPPENS AT HOME

When death occurs at home, you may feel an urgency to do something, but there is no rush.

- With your home care nurse or doctor, develop a plan ahead of time for the process of who is to be contacted at the time of death. Do not call 911 or an emergency response team unless otherwise suggested to you as part of the plan. Usually if an emergency crew is called, they arrive expecting to save a life or give aggressive attempted resuscitation intervention. Emergency ambulance crews are bound by law to do this unless a Do Not Resuscitate order is written by your doctor and communicated to them.

- Each community health care team may have a process and guidelines to follow when an expected death occurs at home. It is best to ask and know about this before your loved one dies.
- Your loved one may have already expressed final wishes and made funeral and other arrangements, or you may need to make arrangements. (see Appendix VIII *Planning Ahead For the Funeral,* page 163). Please remember to reach out if you need support and direction.
- Do not feel that you must call the funeral home immediately after the death. Sometimes friends and family who were not present at death want to come to see the person.
- Be understanding of anyone who chooses to gently hug, caress or bathe the person. These are all normal ways of working through the finality of death.
- Call your home care nurse and family doctor to let them know that death has occurred.
- Ask your funeral home staff and/or your home care nurse how you should take care of and prepare your loved one's body before it leaves the home.

## HOW YOU CAN COMFORT YOURSELF AND LOVED ONES

Remember there is no hurry.

- If you have a spiritual leader and have talked about availability, you may wish to ask that person to be with you and conduct appropriate farewell rituals at the bedside.
- Family and friends may find it helps to gather around your loved one and take a moment to express a prayer, memories or words of appreciation (aloud or silently) for the person's life.
- A farewell gesture of a hug, a kiss or a significant spiritual gesture may help to honour the moment and bring closure.
- Be in physical contact with others if that gives you comfort.
- Do things that calm you, such a having a warm drink or breathing deeply.
- Spend as much time with your loved one as you wish. Take time to say your good-byes.
- Remember, it may or may not be distressing for you or other family members to be present when your loved one is taken to the funeral home. You can decide if you wish to be in or out of the house at that time.

## ARRANGEMENTS AFTER DEATH

Arrangements after a death are emotional tasks that are most often done when you are the least able to think as clearly about such decisions. Choosing to make arrangements in advance can help. (see Appendix VIII Planning Ahead For the Funeral, page 163). When this is done beforehand, there is more time to be more present with family and begin mourning without worrying about organizational details. Your loved one may have also prepared for this and shared wishes with you, which may also make it easier. For other people, making arrangements in advance seems too final and difficult to do. There is no correct or incorrect way to do the planning. It is personal and unique to each person.

## ADVANCE PLANNING OF FINAL ARRANGEMENTS

### What you need to consider

- If you have chosen a funeral home and place of memorial service in advance, this can help with early planning and making arrangements when death occurs.
- Planning in advance often gives you more time to make decisions about the details involved.
- You may save money if you pre-visit or contact several funeral homes to find one that meets your particular needs.
- Pre-paying for a funeral may help lower the costs.
- Your loved one may want to plan a service with you before death occurs.
- Some families choose not to have a service, recognizing their loved one in some other way.

## DECISIONS AFTER DEATH

### What you need to consider

When your loved one dies, there are immediate details that need attention.

## PRACTICAL DETAILS

Several of the following practical aspects of planning may have been decided in advance.

- Family members and close friends should be informed about the death. It may help to have a list with names and numbers already made and some other people assigned to help you with this.

- If flowers and a printed program are to be used, assign someone to arrange for these.
- You may choose to write a newspaper obituary. During this stressful time, it can be easy to make mistakes with details. Be sure to have someone else read the final copy carefully before submitting it.
- If you wish to have donations given to a charity, you need to decide which one. It can be included in the obituary announcement.
- Keep track of cards, visitors and donations so you can acknowledge these at a quieter later time.

## PLANNING A FUNERAL OR MEMORIAL SERVICE

If you have planned a service in advance, you may already have decided about some of the following points. The memorial society, funeral home or another service available in your community can guide you on the details.

- You will need to decide if your loved one is to be buried or cremated.
  - If buried, do you already have a plot you wish to use?
  - If cremated, will the remains be buried, kept or scattered?
  - Sometimes after a cremation, people create a memory place where the ashes are buried and they can go to visit.
- A service can take the form of a funeral, a memorial, a simple graveside or other service.
- Sometimes a bedside service is chosen if direct cremation has been selected. This will be the final opportunity for people to physically see their loved one.
- If you do not have a regular place of worship, consider where a service might be held. Options may include a church, funeral chapel, a community hall or your home.
- Decide on and approach the person you hope to have conducting the service. Depending on the form you choose, it may be a religious or spiritual leader, chaplain, friend, or family member.
- Some people make an audio or video tape of the service. This way, the carefully chosen words can be replayed anytime, and sent to those who could not attend the service. Even family members who attend the funeral often appreciate being able to see or hear it again as they go through the grief and healing process.
- In any planning you do, consider the schedules of people coming from out of town.

## NECESSARY PERSONAL INFORMATION

The District Registrar of Deaths requires the following information about the person who died. You will need this information when you meet with the funeral director. The funeral director will record and forward it to the appropriate government department, along with a Medical Certificate of Death. This information is needed for the funeral director to obtain a death certificate and a permit for burial or cremation.

**NAME:**
LAST NAME (BIRTH/MAIDEN NAME FOR A WOMAN IN QUEBEC) — ALL GIVEN NAMES

**ADDRESS**
HOUSE/APARTMENT # STREET/ROAD — CITY/TOWN — POSTAL CODE

**MARITAL STATUS (MARRIAGE CERTIFICATE MAY BE REQUIRED)**
SINGLE/MARRIED/WIDOWED/DIVORCED/COMMON LAW/CIVIL UNION

| | |
|---|---|
| **MAIDEN NAME** | **OCCUPATION** |
| **BIRTHDATE** *(BIRTH CERTIFICATE MAY BE REQUIRED):* | **AGE** |

| | | |
|---|---|---|
| **BIRTHPLACE** | | |
| CITY/TOWN | PROV/COUNTRY | IF NATIVE, GIVE BAND |

| | |
|---|---|
| **DATE OF DEATH** | **PLACE OF DEATH** |
| **FATHER'S NAME** | |
| **FATHER'S BIRTHPLACE** | |
| **MOTHER'S NAME** | **MOTHER'S MAIDEN NAME** |
| **MOTHER'S BIRTHPLACE** | |

| | | | |
|---|---|---|---|
| **SEX** | **HEIGHT** | **WEIGHT** | **RELIGION** |

**NEXT OF KIN**
NAME

**ADDRESS**
HOUSE/APARTMENT # STREET/ROAD — CITY/TOWN — POSTAL CODE

| | |
|---|---|
| **HEALTH INSURANCE NUMBER** | **SOCIAL INSURANCE NUMBER** |
| **FAMILY DOCTOR** | |

**DOCTOR'S ADDRESS**
HOUSE/APARTMENT # STREET/ROAD — CITY/TOWN — POSTAL CODE

## PLACES TO NOTIFY

1. Contact the funeral director to complete arrangements.

| FUNERAL DIRECTOR | PHONE |
|---|---|

2. Complete the Vital Statistics Guide and take it to your appointment with the funeral director.
3. Contact the Executor/trix, lawyers or notaries involved with the will.

| FUNERAL DIRECTOR | PHONE |
|---|---|
| CO-EXECUTOR | PHONE |

4. Prepare a list of people to be notified. Ask someone to help you with contacting those on the list.

| TELEPHONE HELPER | PHONE |
|---|---|

5. If desired, write an obituary notice to be printed in the newspaper of your choice. This can be costly so you may want to consider its length, how many insertions, and in which newspapers. The funeral director can assist you.
6. If you wish, write or telephone acknowledgement of flowers, cards and donations. Many charitable organizations send thank-you cards to donors and notify the family of any donations received.

| CHARITY | PHONE |
|---|---|

7. Notify Canada/Quebec Pension, banks, landlord or mortgage company, insurance company, utility company, land registry and motor vehicle offices. You will most likely require several copies of the Death Certificate to complete arrangements with them.

| CANADA/QUEBEC PENSION OFFICE | PHONE |
|---|---|
| LANDLORD/ MORTGAGE CO. | PHONE |
| INSURANCE COMPANY | PHONE |
| BANK | PHONE |

## BENEFITS

Most benefits are not automatic, so you must apply for them. Contact:

1. Canada/Quebec Pension Plan Office – you must apply for benefits (lump sum death benefit, survivor's benefits, or dependent children's benefits). The Quebec benefits are almost identical to those of the Canada Pension. You will need your own and the deceased's Social Insurance Numbers (SIN).

| | |
|---|---|
| **YOUR SIN** | **PHONE** |

2. The person's life insurance company/ies (if relevant)

| | |
|---|---|
| **INSURANCE COMPANY** | **PHONE** |
| **INSURANCE COMPANY** | **PHONE** |

3. Private Pension Plans

| | |
|---|---|
| **PENSION PLAN** | **PHONE** |
| **PENSION PLAN** | **PHONE** |

4. Department of Veterans Affairs – If the person served in the Canadian Armed Forces, dependents may be eligible for a pension.

| | |
|---|---|
| **MILITARY ID** | **PHONE** |

5. Any other memberships that have death benefits, such as Union, Canadian Automobile Association/CAA-Quebec, Credit Union/Caisse Populaire, and fraternal orders.

| | |
|---|---|
| **NAME** | **PHONE** |
| **NAME** | **PHONE** |
| **NAME** | **PHONE** |

## OTHER

Contact medical and health people not immediately involved with the person's death.

a) Provincial health insurance – See Appendix VI for your provincial phone number.
b) Supplementary health care coverage – See Appendix VI for your provincial phone number.
c) Contact any clubs, associations, library, magazines, book clubs, etc. of which the person was a member.
d) Contact your car insurance agency. (If registration is in the person's name, you may need new registration). In Quebec, contact the Société de l'assurance-automobile du Québec (SAAQ) Phone: 1-800-361-7620.

# GRIEF

■

When people are trying to adjust to the death of a loved one, it is normal to experience grief. Grief is part of a natural healing process that helps in remembering a loved one and moving forward to adjust to a different life without that person.

## What you need to know

Grieving is an active coping process of re-learning a world which is deeply changed after the death of a loved one. It affects people physically, emotionally, mentally, spiritually and socially. Although there are common emotional experiences in grief (such as initial shock, sadness and anger), everyone grieves in their own unique way, and in their own personal time frame. Grief can be complex and it is influenced by many factors including your past experiences of loss, your relationship with the person who died, the nature and timing of the death itself, your unique personality, coping style, spiritual and religious beliefs, similar losses or stressors, and more.

- Grief may be difficult, stressful and tiring. It is important to know it is not an illness.
- Shock and numbness are often experienced immediately following the death, even when the death is expected.
- Feelings of guilt and a period of thinking "what if" and "if only" is common.
- With the often long journey of progressive illness, it is normal to also feel a sense of relief that your loved one is free of any more suffering.
- Anger is a frequent and normal reaction to death. Often it may be directed toward the person who died. Sometimes it may be aimed at other people and things unrelated to the death. It can range from mild irritability to rage. If you feel angry, find ways to express it in a healthy way. Accept that this is a natural part of grieving.
- You will probably feel a deep sadness and loneliness after the death of a loved one.
- You may try not to think about the death, or distract yourself with other things in order to protect yourself from the pain of grief.
- Everyone grieves differently. There are no quick fixes or set ways to grieve.
- The pain of loss never goes away but lessens over time.

### How grief can affect you physically

You may experience such a wide range of physical symptoms that you begin to think you are ill. These are physical reactions to your grief. They may include:

- tight chest, palpitations.
- shortness of breath.
- diarrhea, constipation, or vomiting.
- crying or sighing.
- lack of energy or weakness.
- dizziness, shivering, or faintness.
- restlessness.
- loss of appetite, overeating.
- trouble sleeping or sleeping too much.
- increased alcohol or drug use.
- reduced sexual drive.
- similar symptoms to what your loved one experienced.

### How grief can affect you mentally

While you are grieving, your mental state may cause many feelings that you have never experienced before. These can include:

- poor concentration.
- confusion, disbelief, "this can't be real."
- constant thoughts about the person.
- daydreaming.
- nightmares or dreams of loss.

### How grief can affect you emotionally

In grief, your emotions may change from hour to hour. This is normal and will settle with time. The range of emotions you might experience include:

- shock, numbness or emptiness.
- withdrawn or explosive moods.
- anger or rage.
- denial or disbelief.
- frustration.
- guilt or regrets.
- pining or yearning.
- sadness, depression, or despair.
- loneliness or isolation.

### How grief can affect you spiritually

No matter what your beliefs, you may go through a period of deep spiritual upheaval. The issues may include:

- blaming life, yourself or the person who has died.
- lack of meaning or purpose in life.
- wanting to die so you can join the dead person.
- continuing to ask "why did this happen?"
- blaming or feeling separation from your spiritual power.

### How grief can affect you socially

When you are grieving, you may feel as if you are alone in understanding the meaning of your loss. You may want the support of others, yet be unwilling to allow them to get close because no one can appreciate what you are going through. Your feelings may include:

- unrealistic expectations of others.
- lack of interest in others' activities.
- withdrawal from people.
- dependence on others.
- fear of being alone.
- feeling out of place with previous friendships.
- rushing into new relationships and surroundings.

## CHILDREN AND GRIEVING

Children do grieve, and this can be in different ways from adults. They may be more likely to express grief through behavior, play and other non-verbal ways (such as art or music) than through talking about it. Their understanding, the way they react and what helps them will vary according to their age, personality, family support system and developmental stage.

- Children feel the sadness of a loss in their family. They may experience heightened fears, worries, and separation anxiety.
- Children may feel anger and guilt about what has happened. It is important to ensure that they know that the death was not their fault.
- Children up to the age of five may have difficulty understanding that death is permanent, as their sense of time is not well developed.
- School-aged children may fear getting sick and dying themselves. If the loved one who died was a parent, they may worry that the other parent will die too.
- Teens will understand better than younger children, though they may not want to talk about the death or their feelings. It is natural for teens to seek support from their peers rather than from the adults in their lives.

### How you can offer comfort and care to children

How parents grieve affects the way their children grieve. People who smile bravely when they are sad confuse children. Adults who acknowledge their feelings are better able to help their children to accept and understand their grief. Certain books may also help children during their grief.

- Include the child in what is happening.
- Tell the truth and give lots of support.
- Listen carefully to the meaning behind what children are saying about their feelings.
- Be honest and give answers in words they understand.
- Reassure children that illness does not always lead to death.
- Remind children that they are loved just as much as ever during your time of grief.
- Tell children that their thoughts and feelings are normal and it is okay to cry.
- Reassure them that others understand their grief.
- Encourage them to express feelings with talking, painting, poetry, puppets and music.
- Try to keep the children's routine as much the same as possible.

## TAKING CARE OF YOURSELF WHEN GRIEVING

It is difficult to anticipate how you will react when death occurs. The important thing to remember is that there are no right or wrong ways to behave.

- Accept your need to grieve and to feel your loss. It is okay to cry and express your sadness.
- Talk about your feelings if this gives you comfort. Choose someone you are comfortable with who is a good listener.
- Take your time in resuming your regular activities. Be patient with yourself when you are confused or forgetful.
- Look after yourself physically. Eat well, exercise and get lots of rest. Poor nutrition leaves you at risk of health problems.
- Do something nice for yourself each day.
- Explore what life and death mean to you.
- Do not isolate yourself. Meet with friends, talk about your loss, and mention your loved one by name.
- Be careful when driving. Poor concentration and 'blanking out' can be hazardous.
- Slow down and let some responsibilities go for a time. Low energy is to be expected.

- Restrict drugs and alcohol. They can depress your ability to think clearly and postpone natural grieving.
- Recognize that palpitations, digestive problems, chest pains, shortness of breath are all normal reactions to grief. However, it is still important to contact your doctor and have them checked out.
- Make time to do the things you enjoy, and to strive to still live the best you can each day.
- Try to focus on several positive things each day.
- Take time to be alone when you need it.
- If prayer is a part of your daily life, continue to pray. Be gentle with yourself if it takes a while before you start to pray again. Let others continue to carry you in their prayers.
- Check to see if your community has grief support groups, information sessions or support services if you feel you need to reach out for extra information, understanding and help.
- Seek resources for suggestions that you and your loved ones might find helpful during this time of grief.
- On special occasions (such as Christmas, Easter, Valentine's, Mother's or Father's day) or times that are uniquely special to you (such as anniversaries, special trips, and personal moments), grief may come on strong again. Take time to remember your loved one by telling friends and family what you need and asking for their support. Celebrate that special occasion. Take the time to do small somethings in your loved one's memory such as lighting a candle, planting a flower, or making a memorial donation.
- Strive to be gentle, kind and patient with yourself and those around you.
- Remind yourself that the days will be different now, and that you and your family are just beginning to learn how to cope and adjust with what will be different.
- Remember to take it one moment at a time.

## HOW LONG GRIEF MAY LAST

It is hard to say how long a person will experience intense grief. People mistakenly think you should be back to normal in just a few months. This is not the case.

- Many people find that grief comes and goes in waves for a long time.
- After several months intense feelings may begin to ease.
- It may take a long time before you begin to feel more balanced, have the energy to build new interests or find that life begins to have some meaning again.
- Over time, coping gets easier and confidence begins to return.
- It may take you a long time to return to places or things you once enjoyed together before the death.
- As you strive to develop a new and different life, it can take time to feel you can live fully again without your loved one.
- Even when you think you are over your grief, feelings may be triggered by such things as dates, occasions, places, songs, films or poems.
- Know that your feelings of grief do fluctuate and ease with time. Remind yourself that this is normal and a part of the ongoing healing process.

### IMPORTANT POINTS

*Remember to find healthy ways to cope. Ask yourself what has helped before in facing past difficulties or losses, and draw upon those methods now. If or when you find such strategies no longer help, be honest with yourself as you answer the following questions:*

**Since the death are you:**

- *always bad tempered and angry?*
- *busy all the time, restless or unable to keep your mind on what you should be doing?*
- *afraid of getting too close to other people for fear of facing loss again?*
- *finding that you keep going over and over the same things in your mind?*
- *unable to get rid of guilt about what you did or did not do before the person died?*
- *feeling numb and alone all of the time?*
- *thinking more about your own death?*
- *doing things that may prove harmful to yourself, such as drinking a lot of alcohol, using more medications, or driving carelessly?*
- *having frequent thoughts of suicide?*
- *more fearful for no good reason?*

*Grief can develop into a clinical depression that needs professional help. If you answered yes to any of the above questions, and the issues continue more than one year after the death, please see your doctor or health care professional for advice.*

# FINAL THOUGHTS

■

For some caregivers of people with a progressive illness, grief may have been experienced before the death. You may hear the words "anticipatory grief" used to describe it. The death itself may bring a sense of closure and healing may have already begun. For others, the process of grief may take longer. For everyone, healing can take many forms as life gradually returns to a new normal.

- There may be a tremendous sense of relief that the suffering of the person is over.
- As you have time to reflect, you may review and see many examples of courage and dignity that took place in the midst of such a difficult time.
- You may feel a stronger bond with family and friends who have supported you.
- Contentment and happy feelings may begin to return.
- You may feel as though you can start a new life with new experiences.
- You can choose to live life to the fullest and carry on, as your loved one would have done.

Always remember that you will carry the memory of your loved one in your heart. That person may have played an important role in your life. Take comfort in knowing that by supporting them in the final stages of life, you shared in the most loving final gift of comfort, compassion and care.

> *"I know for certain that we never lose the people we love, even to death. They continue to participate in every act, thought and decision we make. Their love leaves an indelible imprint in our memories. We find comfort in knowing that our lives have been enriched by having shared their love."*
>
> *—Leo Buscaglia*

CHAPTER

# 5

# BOOKS AND OTHER RESOURCES THAT MAY BE HELPFUL

# WRITTEN MATERIALS

■

Baker, Tom. (2008). | ***So You've Been Appointed Executor.***
Canada: Self-Counsel Press.

Buckman, R. (1988). | ***I Don't Know What To Say.***
Toronto, ON: Key Porter Books Limited.

Byock, I. (1997). | ***Dying Well.*** | New York, NY: Riverhead Books.

Callanan, M. & Kelley, P. (1997). | ***Final Gifts: Understanding the special awareness, needs, and communications of the dying.***
Bantam Books Canada, Incorporated.

Canadian Cancer Society. (1985). | ***Taking Time: Support for people living with cancer and people who care about them.*** | Bethesda, MD: National Cancer Institute. [Pamphlet: to obtain contact Canadian Cancer Society.]

Canadian Cancer Society. (1983). | ***Nutrition for people with cancer.***
Toronto, ON: Department of Nutrition at the Ontario Cancer Institute, Princess Margaret Hospital and the Canadian Cancer Society.

Canadian Hospice Palliative Care Association and The GlaxoSmithKline Foundation (2002). ***Living Lessons: a guide for caregivers.***
Toronto, ON. GlaxoSmithKline Inc.

Canadian Hospice Palliative Care Association and The GlaxoSmithKline Foundation (2002). | ***Influencing Change: A patient and caregiver advocacy guide.*** | Toronto, ON. GlaxoSmithKline Inc.

D'Aprix, Dr. Amy. (2008). | ***From Surviving to Thriving: Transforming your caregiver journey.*** | Canada: Second Life Press.

Deachman, M., & Howell, D. (1991). | ***Supportive Care at Home: A guide for terminally ill patients and their families.*** | Markham, ON: Knoll Pharmaceuticals Canada [Pamphlet: to obtain contact Knoll Pharmaceuticals Canada, Markham, ON].

Decter, Michael and Francesca Grosso. (2008). | ***Navigating Canada's Health Care: A user's guide to getting what you need.***
Toronto: Penguin Canada.

Dyregov, Atle. | ***Grief in Children: a handbook for adults.*** (2008)
Philadelphia, PA. Jessica Kingsley Publishers.

Emswiler, James P. and Mary Ann Emswiler. (2000).
***Guiding your Child Through Grief.*** | New York: Bantam Books.

Golden, S. (1988). ***Nursing a Loved One at Home: A care giver's guide.***
Philadelphia, PA: Running Press.

Gordon, Michael. (2010). | ***Moments that Matter: Cases in ethical eldercare.*** | Indiana: iUniverse.

Grollman, E. A. (1987). | ***In Sickness and in Health: How to cope when your loved one is ill.*** | Boston: Beacon Press.

Grollman, E. A. (1993). | ***Straight Talk About Death for Teenagers: How to cope with losing someone you love.*** | Boston: Beacon Press.

Grollman, E. A. (1976). | ***Talking About Death: A dialogue between parent and child.*** | Boston: Beacon Press.

Jevne, R. F. (1994). | ***The Voice of Hope: Heard across the heart of life.***
San Diego, CA: Lura Media.

Jevne, R. F. (1991). | ***It All Begins With Hope: Patients, caregivers & the bereaved speak out.*** | San Diego, CA: Lura Media.

Jevne, R. F., & Levitan, A. (1989). | ***No Time for Nonsense: Self-help for the seriously ill.*** | San Diego, CA: Lura Media.

Kübler-Ross, E. and David Kessler. (2005). | ***On Grief and Grieving: Finding the Meaning of Grief Through the Five Stages of Loss.*** | New York, NY. Scribner.

Kuhl, David. | ***What Dying People Want: Practical wisdom for the end of life.*** | Canada: Public Affairs.

Latimer, E. J. (1996). ***Easing the Hurt: A handbook of comfort for families and friends of people who are seriously ill.*** | Hamilton, ON: Purdue Frederick. [Pamphlet: to obtain contact Purdue Frederick Inc., 575 Granite Court, Pickering, Ontario, L1W 3W8.]

McFarlane, R., & Bashe, P. (1998). | ***The Complete Bedside Companion: A no-nonsense guide to caring for the seriously ill.*** | New York: Simon & Schuster.

Murray, Katherine. (2009). | ***Essentials in Palliative Care: a resource for caregivers.*** | Canada: Life and Death Matters.

O'Rourke, Michelle, & Eugene Dufour. (2012). | ***Embracing the End of Life: Help for those who accompany the dying.*** | Canada: Novalis.

Paulus, Trina. (1973/1997). | ***Hope for the Flowers.***
New Jersey: Paulist Press.

Pinchot, Laura. (2010). | ***Help Wanted: Caregiver: A Guide to Helping your loved one cope with serious illness.*** | United States. Oncology Nursing Society.

Rando, T. A. (1991). | ***How to Go on Living When Someone You Love Dies.*** | New York: Bantam Books.

Schonfeld, David and Marcia Quackenbush. | ***After a Loved One Dies – How Children Grieve: and how parents and other adults can support them.*** (2009). New York, NY. New York Life Foundation.

Siegel, B. S. (1990). | ***Love, Medicine & Miracles: Lessons learned about self-healing from a surgeon's experience with exceptional patients.***
New York: Harper Perennial.

Siegel, B. S. (1989). | ***Peace, Love & Healing: Body mind communication and the path to self-healing: An exploration.*** | New York: Harper & Row.

van Bommel, H. (1999). | ***Caring for Loved Ones at Home.***
To obtain book, contact Resources Supporting Family and Community Legacies Inc. Scarborough, On.

White, P. (Ed.). (1986). | ***Home Care of the Hospice Patient: An informational/ instructional booklet for caregivers in the home.***
Chicago, IL: Rush-Presbyterian- St. Luke's Medical Centre. [Pamphlet: to obtain contact Purdue Frederick Inc., 575 Granite Court Pickering, Ontario, L1W 3W8.]

Wolfelt, Alan. (2004). | ***Understanding Grief: Ten essential touchstones for finding hope and healing your heart.*** | Colorado: Companion Press.

Wolfelt, Alan (2001). | ***Healing a Teenager's Grieving Heart: 100 practical ideas for families, friends and caregivers.*** | Colorado: Companion Press.

Wolfelt, Alan (2001). | ***Healing the Bereaved Child.***
Colorado: Companion Press.

# BOOKS TO HELP GRIEVING CHILDREN

■

Buscaglia, L. (1983). | ***The Fall of Freddie the Leaf.***
New Jersey: Holt, Rinehart & Winston.

Gobie, P. (1993). | ***Beyond the Ridge.*** | New York Aladdin Paperbacks.

Gootman, M., Espeland, P, & Prothrow-Smith, D.
(1994). | ***When a Friend Dies.*** | Free Spirit Publishers.

Grollman, E. (1993). | ***Straight Talk about Death for Teenagers.*** | United States: Beacon Press.

Grollman, E. (1991). | ***Talking about Death.*** | United States: Beacon Press.

Hanson, Warren. (1997). | ***The Next Place.***
United States of America: Waldman House Press.

Heegaard, Marge Eaton. (2002). | ***Beyond the Rainbow: a workbook for children in the advanced stages of a very serious illness.***
Minnesota: Fairview Press.

Mellonie, Bryan. (1983). | ***Lifetimes: The beautiful way to explain death to children.*** | United States: Bantam Books.

Mills, Joyce C. & Cary Pillo (2003). | ***Gentle Willow: A story for children about dying.*** | United States of America: Magination Press.

Vigna, J. & Levine, A. (1991). | ***Saying Goodbye to Daddy.***
United States: A. Whitman.

Winsch, Jane Loretta and Pamela T. Keating. | ***After the Funeral (1995).***
USA: Paulist Press.

# INTERNET RESOURCES

■

After Giving | *www.aftergiving.com*

Alberta Health Services Caregiver Centre | *www.albertahealthservices.ca/3731.asp*

Alberta Hospice Palliative Care Association | *ahpca.ca*

Alexandra Kennedy | *www.alexandrakennedy.com*

BC Caregiver Network's Information Package for Family Caregivers
*thefamilycaregiver.com/bc/caregiving/caregiving.php*

Bereaved Families Online Support Centre | *www.bereavedfamilies.net*

Bereavement | *www.bereavementselfhelp.victoria.bc.ca*

British Columbia Hospice Palliative Care Association | *www.bchpca.org*

Capital Health Regional Palliative Care Program
*palliative.org/NewPC/Resources/general_resources.html*

Caregivers' Aspirations, Realities and Expectations Tool | *tinyurl.com/kffjnbd*

Caregiver Connect | *www.caregiver-connect.ca*

Caregiver Network (Canadian) | *www.caregiver.ca*

Caregiver Self-Assessment Guide | *tinyurl.com/n59mbzs*

Caregiver Survival Resources (American) | *www.caregiver911.com*

Caring to the End of Life | *www.caringtotheend.ca*

Canadian Cancer Society's *If you're a Caregiver*
*www.cancer.ca/en/cancer-information/cancer-journey/*
*if-you-re-a-caregiver/?region=mb*

Cancer Chat Canada: Caregiver Support | *cancerchatcanada.ca*

Canadian Funeral Home Directory offering various support resources
*www.generations.on.ca./index.html*

Canadian Hospice Palliative Care Association | *www.chpca.net*

Canadian Virtual Hospice | *www.virtualhospice.ca*

Center for Grieving Children | *www.cgcmaine.org*

Compassion Books – an online source of over 400 books for grieving children and adults | *www.compassionbooks.com*

Crisis, Grief and Healing | *www.webhealing.com*

Dying Well (American) | *www.dyingwell.com*

ElderWeb (American) | *www.elderweb.com*

Family Caregiver Alliance | *www.caregiver.org*

Family Caregivers Network Society | *www.fcns-caregiving.org*

Fernside (Support for grieving children and families) | *www.fernside.org*

Genesis Bereavement Centres | *www.genesis-resources.com*

Grief, Loss & Recovery | *www.grieflossrecovery.com*

Grieving Children | *www.grievingchildren.com*

Hospice and Palliative Care Manitoba | *www.manitobahospice.ca*

Hospice Palliative Care Ontario | *www.hpco.ca*

Hospice Palliative Care Prince Edward Island | *hospicepei.ca*

Hospice Net, For Patients and Families Facing Life-Threatening Illness
*www.hospicenet.org*

Journey of Hearts | *www.journeyofhearts.org*

Living Lessons | *www.living-lessons.org*

Mourning Star Centre (Support for grieving children and families)
*www.mourningstar.org*

New Brunswick Hospice Palliative Care Association
*www.nbhpca-aspnb.ca*

Nova Scotia Hospice Palliative Care Association | *www.nshpca.ca*

Family Hospice Care | *www.legacies.ca*

Réseau de soins palliatifs du Québec | *www.aqsp.org*

Saskatchewan Hospice Palliative Care Association | *www.saskpalliativecare.org*

Seniors BC | *www.seniorsBC.ca*

What Do I Do Now? (Guidance for requirement after a death)
*www.nsnet.org/bereaved*

Wisdom of the World (Varied resources) | *www.gracefulpassages.com*

# REFERENCES USED IN PREPARATION OF THIS BOOK

■

Berry, L. & Schneider, T. (1997). | ***What Do I Do Now?*** | Red Deer, AB: Eventide Funeral Chapels.

Buckman, R. (1988). | ***I Don't Know What to Say.*** | Toronto, ON: Key Porter Books Limited.

Canadian Cancer Society. (1983). | ***Nutrition for People with Cancer.*** Toronto, ON: Department of Nutrition at the Ontario Cancer Institute, Princess Margaret Hospital and the Canadian Cancer Society.

Canadian Cancer Society. (1985). | ***Taking Time: Support for people living with cancer and people who care about them.*** | Bethesda, MD: National Cancer Institute.

Canadian Palliative Care Association and the Canadian Association for Community Care. (1998). | ***Training Manual for Support Workers in Palliative Care.*** Ottawa, ON: Canadian Palliative Care Association.

Cantwell, P., MacKay, S., Macmillan, K., Turco, S., McKinnon, S., Read-Paul, L. (1988). | ***99 Common Questions (and Answers) about Palliative Care: a nurse's handbook.*** | Edmonton, AB: Regional Palliative Care Program, Capital Health Authority.

Cassileth, B.R. (Ed.). (1986). | ***Caring for the Terminally Ill Patient at Home: A guide for family caregivers.*** | University of Pennsylvania Cancer Centre Hospice and Homecare Program.

Capital Health Home Care (1996) | ***Changing Your Infusion Tubing and Preloading a Single Insulin.***

Deachman, M., & Howell, D. (1991). | ***Supportive Care at Home: A guide for terminally ill patients and their families.*** | Markham, ON: Knoll Pharmaceuticals Canada.

Baker, Tom. (2008). | ***So You've Been Appointed Executor.*** | Canada: Self-Counsel Press.

Byock, I. (1997). | ***Dying Well.*** | New York, NY: Riverhead Books.

Callanan, M. & Kelley, P. (1997). | ***Final Gifts: Understanding the special awareness, needs, and communications of the dying.*** | Bantam Books Canada, Incorporated.

Canadian Hospice Palliative Care Association and The GlaxoSmithKline Foundation (2002). | ***Living Lessons: a Guide for Caregivers.*** | Toronto, ON. GlaxoSmithKline Inc.

Canadian Hospice Palliative Care Association and The GlaxoSmithKline Foundation (2002). | ***Influencing Change: A patient and caregiver advocacy guide.*** | Toronto, ON. GlaxoSmithKline Inc.

D'Aprix, Dr. Amy. (2008). | ***From Surviving to Thriving: Transforming your caregiver journey.*** | Canada: Second Life Press.

Deachman, M., & Howell, D. (1991). | ***Supportive Care at Home: A guide for terminally ill patients and their families.*** | Markham, ON: Knoll Pharmaceuticals Canada [Pamphlet: to obtain contact Knoll Pharmaceuticals Canada, Markham, ON.

Decter, Michael and Francesca Grosso. (2008). |
***Navigating Canada's Health Care: A user's guide to getting what you need.***
Toronto: Penguin Canada.

Dyregov, Atle. | ***Grief in Children: a handbook for adults.*** | (2008) Philadelphia, PA. Jessica Kingsley Publishers.

Emswiler, James P. and Mary Ann Emswiler. (2000). | ***Guiding your Child Through Grief.*** | New York: Bantam Books

Golden, S. (1988). | ***Nursing a Loved One at Home: A care giver's guide.*** Philadelphia, PA: Running Press.

Gordon, Michael. (2010). | ***Moments that Matter: Cases in ethical eldercare.*** Indiana: iUniverse.

Grollman, E. A. (1987). | ***In Sickness and in Health: How to cope when your loved one is ill.*** | Boston: Beacon Press.

Grollman, E. A. (1993). | ***Straight Talk about Death for Teenagers: How to cope with losing someone you love.*** | Boston: Beacon Press.

Grollman, E. A. (1976). | ***Talking about Death: A dialogue between parent and child.*** | Boston: Beacon Press.

Jevne, R. F. (1994). | ***The Voice of Hope: Heard across the heart of life.*** San Diego, CA: Lura Media.

Jevne, R. F. (1991). | ***It All Begins with Hope: Patients, caregivers & the bereaved speak out.*** | San Diego, CA: Lura Media.

Jevne, R. F., & Levitan, A. (1989). | ***No Time for Nonsense: Self-help for the seriously ill.*** | San Diego, CA: Lura Media.

Kübler-Ross, E. and David Kessler. (2005). | ***On Grief and Grieving: Finding the meaning of grief through the five stages of loss.*** New York, NY. Scribner.

Kuhl, David. | ***What Dying People Want: Practical wisdom for the end of life.*** | Canada: Public Affairs.

Latimer, E. J. (1996). | ***Easing the Hurt: A handbook of comfort for families and friends of people who are seriously ill.*** | Hamilton, ON: Purdue Frederick. [Pamphlet: to obtain contact Purdue Frederick Inc., 575 Granite Court, Pickering, Ontario, L1W 3W8.

McFarlane, R., & Bashe, P. (1998). | ***The Complete Bedside Companion: A no-nonsense guide to caring for the seriously ill.*** | New York: Simon & Schuster.

Murray, Katherine. (2009). | ***Essentials in Palliative Care: a resource for caregivers.*** | Canada: Life and Death Matters.

O'Rourke, Michelle, & Eugene Dufour. (2012). | ***Embracing the End of Life: Help for those who accompany the dying.*** | Canada: Novalis.

Paulus, Trina. (1973/1997). | ***Hope for the Flowers.*** New Jersey: Paulist Press.

Pinchot, Laura. (2010). | ***Help Wanted: Caregiver: A guide to helping your loved one cope with serious illness.*** | United States. Oncology Nursing Society.

Rando, T. A. (1991). | ***How to Go on Living When Someone You Love Dies.*** | New York: Bantam Books.

Schonfeld, David and Marcia Quackenbush. | ***After a Loved One Dies – How Children Grieve: and how parents and other adults can support them.*** (2009). New York, NY. New York Life Foundation.

Siegel, B. S. (1990). | ***Love, Medicine & Miracles: Lessons learned about self-healing from a surgeon's experience with exceptional patients.*** | New York: Harper Perennial.

Siegel, B. S. (1989). | ***Peace, Love & Healing: Body mind communication and the path to self-healing: An exploration.*** | New York: Harper & Row.

van Bommel, H. (1999). | ***Caring for Loved Ones at Home.***
To obtain book, contact Resources Supporting Family and Community Legacies Inc. Scarborough, On.

White, P. (Ed.). (1986). | ***Home Care of the Hospice Patient: An informational/ instructional booklet for caregivers in the home.***
Chicago, IL: Rush-Presbyterian- St. Luke's Medical Centre.
[Pamphlet: to obtain contact Purdue Frederick Inc., 575 Granite Court Pickering, Ontario, L1W 3W8.

Wolfelt, Alan. (2004). | ***Understanding Grief: Ten essential touchstones for finding hope and healing your heart.*** | Colorado: Companion Press.

Wolfelt, Alan (2001). | ***Healing a Teenager's Grieving Heart: 100 practical ideas for families, friends and caregivers.*** | Colorado: Companion Press.

Wolfelt, Alan (2001). | ***Healing the Bereaved Child.*** | Colorado: Companion Press.

# APPENDIX I
# FINANCIAL AID

■

There are many resources available that may help you financially while you are caring for a loved one who is terminally ill. Ask a member of your health care team for advice about the following possibilities. Also see Appendix VI, where provincial contacts for financial aid are provided.

### Canada Pension or Quebec Pension Plan

A disability pension is payable to anyone under 65 who has contributed to the Canada or Quebec Pension Plan for a specified period of time, and has a severe and prolonged disability.

Phone: 1-800-277-9914 (for CPP-English) | 1-800-277-9915 (for CPP-French)
1-800-363-3911 or website www.rrq.gouv.qc.ca (for QPP)

### Guaranteed Income Supplement

You may be eligible for this supplement, if you are over 65 and depending on your income. For instance, you would most likely qualify if your only income is the Old Age Security.

Phone: 1-800-277-9914

### Old Age Security

If you or the person you are caring for turns 65 during this period of palliative care, be aware the Old Age Security will not come automatically. An application should be submitted six months before the 65th birthday. You may need to help begin this process.

Phone: 1-800-277-9914 (English) | 1-800-277-9915 (French)
Régime de pensions du Canada, 1-800-277-9915

In Quebec province, you can qualify for the "Régie des Rentes du Québec" if you have worked in the province during your life and if you have paid taxes to the Quebec government. Phone: Régie des Rentes du Québec (418) 643-5185 ou www.rrq.gouv.qc.ca

### Social Assistance

If you receive social assistance, you may qualify for financial help with medical expenses, prescriptions and special health needs. If you do not already receive social assistance, but do have a low income, you may also be able to get help with certain expenses. The phone number of the office closest to your home will be listed in the phone book under a provincial listing for Human Resources, or see Appendix VI for your provincial phone number.

### Employment Insurance

You may qualify for Employment Insurance if you have made contributions during the last 52 weeks. The requirements vary depending on where you live in Canada and the unemployment rate in your economic region at the time of filing your claim. Call the number below for information about whether or not you qualify.

Phone: 1-800-206-7218 | 1-800-808-6352 (Quebec)

### Department of Veterans Affairs (DVA)

If your loved one is a veteran, you may be eligible for:

- an attendance allowance for care given during the illness.
- a disability pension.
- equipment and home alterations.

Contact a DVA counsellor to discuss your situation. You will need to know the person's service number.

Phone: 1-800-665-3420 | 1-800-291-0471(Quebec)

### Private Insurance and Supplementary Health Care Plans

Check the documents you have for insurance and extended health care coverage. Benefits covered may include ambulance, nursing care, Home Support Aide, medications, and oxygen.

### Palliative Care Drug Coverage

Some provinces subsidize the cost of certain medications used by a person receiving palliative care at home. A doctor must confirm on an application that palliative care is being given. When the application is accepted, the required medications can be obtained at your local pharmacy. (See page 154 Appendix VI - *Provincial Contacts for Further Medical, Legal and Financial* to find out if this is available in your province, and for the contact phone number.)

### Life Insurance Policies

If a family member has a serious illness, it may be possible to apply to have your premiums waived without affecting the policy itself. This requires a written application and medical proof of illness.

**Associations, Lodges and Unions**

Check with lodges or other organizations to which the person belongs to see if they provide financial help during a member's illness.

**Canadian Cancer Society and Fondation québecoise du cancer (in Quebec)**

These groups provide financial help with certain medications. There is also assistance with transportation and accommodation. There is a means test to determine eligibility for these programs. Call the numbers listed in your telephone book or

Phone: 1-888-939-3333 (Canada) | 1-877-336-4443 (Quebec)

**Canada Customs and Revenue Agency and Ministère du Revenu du Québec**

When a person has been disabled for an extended time, there may be income tax deductions for that person, dependents and medical expenses. Residents of Quebec should contact both departments.

Phone: 1-800-959-8281 (Canada) | 1 800 267-6299 (Quebec)

**Supplementary Income Programs for Handicapped Persons**

Some provinces provide financial help to adults with severe and permanent disabilities. The amount of money people receive depends on their income. These are not medical programs. People receive assistance if the disability is permanent, meaning they have exhausted all opportunities for rehabilitation, training and work. See Appendix VI for a phone number if this program exists in your province.

**Last Post Fund**

If your loved one left no money and/or was on a war pension, and was a veteran of World War I or II or the Korean Campaign, burial costs may be covered by the Last Post Fund. Any branch of the Royal Canadian Legion (ask for the Service Officer) or the Department of Veterans Affairs can assist you, or the Funeral Director will complete the application for you if you supply the regimental number. See Appendix VI for a provincial listing for the Last Post Fund and contact them before funeral arrangements are made. Federally, a website is *www.lastpostfund.ca* or e-mail at *info@lastpostfund.ca*.

**Special Needs Assistance for Seniors**

Some provinces have a program that provides financial assistance to low income seniors who are experiencing financial difficulties. See Appendix VI for a phone number if this program exists in your province.

# APPENDIX II
# LEGAL AFFAIRS

■

Sometimes it is necessary for one person to act on behalf of another. Three categories of legally binding documents allow the care of an incapacitated person. These documents are enduring power of attorney, guardianship and trusteeship. A fourth category is a personal directive. This is not legally binding but is a statement of a person's wishes.

## Enduring Power of Attorney

An enduring power of attorney is a document that appoints a person to act financially on behalf of someone else who is either physically or mentally incapacitated. A power of attorney should be prepared far in advance of being needed as a safeguard. It is obtained through a lawyer or notary. The person giving the permission must be of sound mind, alert and able to make decisions. Otherwise, the person acting on the power of attorney order is acting without authority. The advantage of the power of attorney is that it gives a dying person the chance to decide who will be managing financial affairs.

## Guardianship

This order is granted by the courts under the Dependent Adults Act. When a person is not able to make decisions such as where to live, health care and daily needs, guardianship permits another person to make these decisions. The guardian is required to decide in the best interest of the person, to encourage independence and to act in the least restrictive manner possible.

## Trusteeship

This is an order under the Dependent Adults Act that gives a person permission to handle the financial affairs of another. The trustee can assume control when someone's mental condition prevents sound decision-making. Legal authority is given to manage, handle, administer, sell and dispose of assets, just as the person could have done. Restrictions may be imposed by the judge and the trustee must file a full inventory and account of assets and liabilities.

A Trustee and a Guardian may both be needed for the same person if the ability to make decisions about daily living and about finances is impaired. To obtain a Trustee or Guardianship order, the assistance of a solicitor is required and a medical report must be filed with the court.

### Old Age Security Trusteeship (Limited Power of Attorney)

This type of trusteeship is for handling cheques for someone else. It allows an appointed person to cash or deposit cheques for another. Cheques may not be written on the account nor funds withdrawn.

### Personal Directive (Living Will)

A personal directive states a person's wishes about medical care if that person is not able to make the decisions. While it is not a legal document, it is intended to ensure that the individual's rights are honoured. Details of a personal directive need to be discussed fully with both your family doctor and immediate family members. Most provincial governments have produced pamphlets to help you write this document. See Appendix VII for a phone number if this type of help exists in your province.

### Mandate in Case of Incapacity (Quebec only)

This document is fully binding, provided a person has been declared incompetent by the provincial court. This finding requires supportive documentation from professionals such as psychiatrists and social workers. (See page 159 for contact information to learn more details about this document).

For further information about the above topics, ask a member of your health care team.

## APPENDIX III

# HOME MEDICATION SCHEDULE

■

| DATE | NAME OF MEDICATION | DOSE | HOW TAKEN | PURPOSE | 12 MIDNIGHT | 2 AM | 4 AM | 6 AM | 8 AM | 10 AM | 12 NOON | 2 PM | 4 PM | 6 PM | 8 PM | 10 PM |
|---|---|---|---|---|---|---|---|---|---|---|---|---|---|---|---|---|
| | | | | | | | | | | | | | | | | |
| | | | | | | | | | | | | | | | | |
| | | | | | | | | | | | | | | | | |
| | | | | | | | | | | | | | | | | |
| | | | | | | | | | | | | | | | | |
| | | | | | | | | | | | | | | | | |
| | | | | | | | | | | | | | | | | |
| | | | | | | | | | | | | | | | | |
| | | | | | | | | | | | | | | | | |
| | | | | | | | | | | | | | | | | |
| | | | | | | | | | | | | | | | | |
| | | | | | | | | | | | | | | | | |
| | | | | | | | | | | | | | | | | |
| | | | | | | | | | | | | | | | | |
| | | | | | | | | | | | | | | | | |
| | | | | | | | | | | | | | | | | |
| | | | | | | | | | | | | | | | | |
| | | | | | | | | | | | | | | | | |

## APPENDIX IV
# SYMPTOM ASSESSMENT SCALE

Circle the number that best describes:

| | | | | | | | | | | | | |
|---|---|---|---|---|---|---|---|---|---|---|---|---|
| **NO PAIN** | 0 | 1 | 2 | 3 | 4 | 5 | 6 | 7 | 8 | 9 | 10 | **WORST POSSIBLE PAIN** |
| **NOT TIRED** | 0 | 1 | 2 | 3 | 4 | 5 | 6 | 7 | 8 | 9 | 10 | **WORST POSSIBLE TIREDNESS** |
| **NOT NAUSEATED** | 0 | 1 | 2 | 3 | 4 | 5 | 6 | 7 | 8 | 9 | 10 | **WORST POSSIBLE NAUSEA** |
| **NOT DEPRESSED** | 0 | 1 | 2 | 3 | 4 | 5 | 6 | 7 | 8 | 9 | 10 | **WORST POSSIBLE DEPRESSION** |
| **NOT DROWSY** | 0 | 1 | 2 | 3 | 4 | 5 | 6 | 7 | 8 | 9 | 10 | **WORST POSSIBLE DROWSINESS** |
| **NOT ANXIOUS** | 0 | 1 | 2 | 3 | 4 | 5 | 6 | 7 | 8 | 9 | 10 | **WORST POSSIBLE ANXIETY** |
| **BEST APPETITE** | 0 | 1 | 2 | 3 | 4 | 5 | 6 | 7 | 8 | 9 | 10 | **WORST POSSIBLE APPETITE** |
| **BEST FEELING OF WELLBEING** | 0 | 1 | 2 | 3 | 4 | 5 | 6 | 7 | 8 | 9 | 10 | **WORST POSSIBLE FEELING OF WELLBEING** |
| **NO SHORTNESS OF BREATH** | 0 | 1 | 2 | 3 | 4 | 5 | 6 | 7 | 8 | 9 | 10 | **SHORTNESS OF BREATH** |
| **OTHER PROBLEM** | 0 | 1 | 2 | 3 | 4 | 5 | 6 | 7 | 8 | 9 | 10 | |

Mark on these pictures where it is that you hurt:

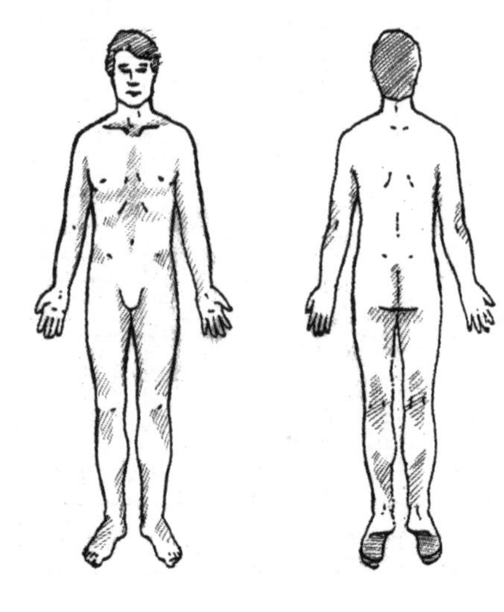

## APPENDIX V
# BREAKTHROUGH MEDICATION CHART

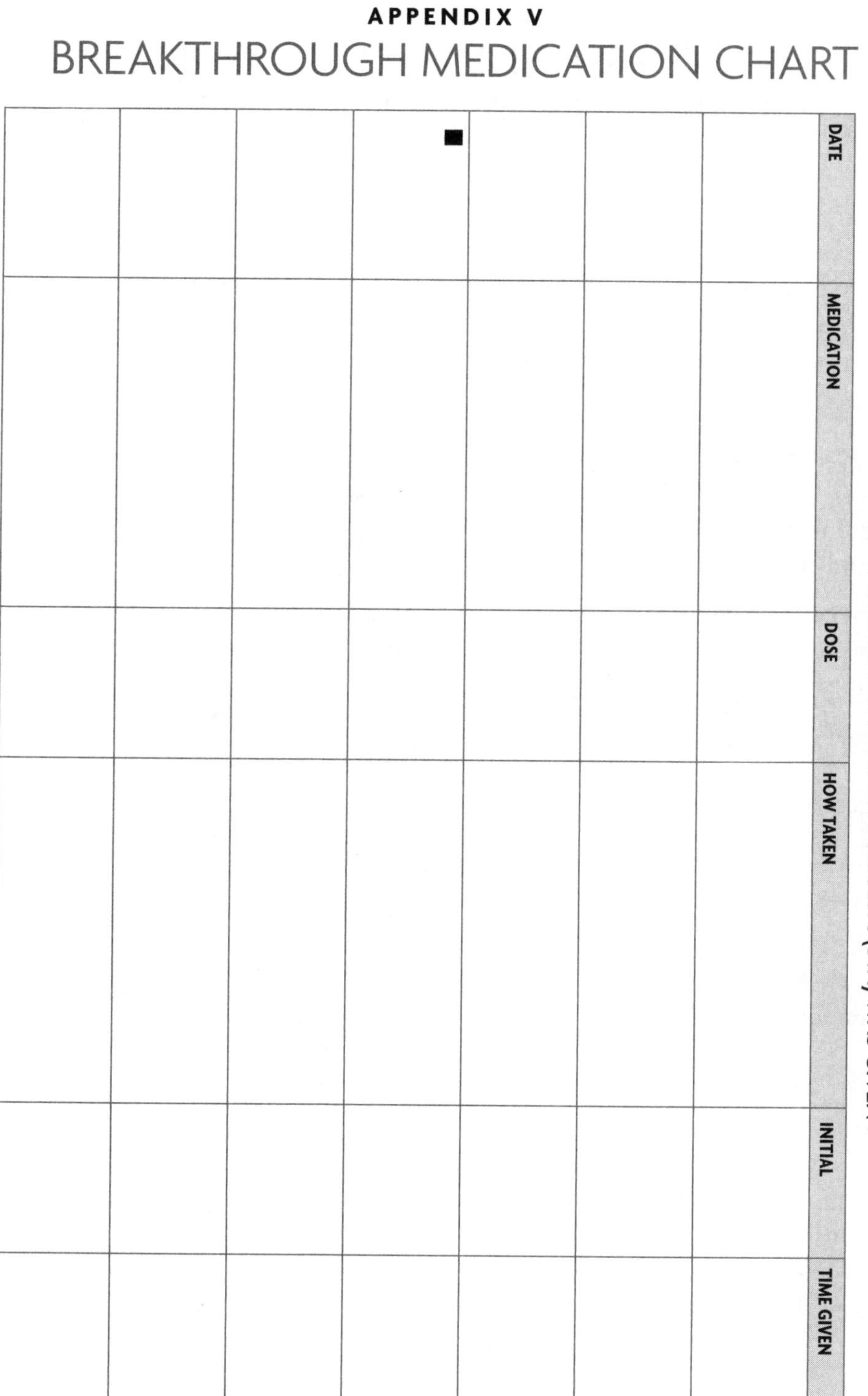

| DATE | MEDICATION | DOSE | HOW TAKEN | INITIAL | TIME GIVEN |
|---|---|---|---|---|---|
| | | | | | |
| | | | | | |
| | | | | | |
| | | | | | |
| | | | | | |
| | | | | | |
| | | | | | |

WRITE IN WHEN THE BREAKTHROUGH ANALGESIC (BTA) WAS GIVEN

## APPENDIX VI

# FURTHER MEDICAL, LEGAL AND FINANCIAL PROVINCIAL CONTACTS

■

The resources listed in this appendix are to help those who already have an established palliative care contact. They are intended to complement the information the home care nurse can provide. If you do not have a palliative care support team and want further information, contact your family doctor.

## ALBERTA

### Provincial Health Care Insurance

**Alberta Health Care Insurance Commission**

Call toll-free Feedback Line (from anywhere in Alberta): 310-4455

### Income Support

**Alberta Employment, Immigration and Industry**

Toll-free in Alberta:
1-866-477-8589
Edmonton: 780-644-1364

### Aids to Daily Living

**Alberta Aids to Daily Living**

Phone: 780-427-2631
or 780-427-0731
Toll-free 310-000 and ask for one of the above numbers.

### Palliative Care Drug Coverage

**Alberta Health and Wellness**
Phone: Edmonton, 780-427-1432
Toll-free 310-0000 and input 780-427-1432

### Supplementary Income Programs for Handicapped Persons

**Assured Income for the Severely Handicapped (AISH)**

Phone: Edmonton, 780-415-6300
Calgary, 403-297-8511
Toll-free 310-0000 and ask for one of the above numbers.

**Last Post Fund**
Phone: Edmonton,
780-495-3766
Toll-free: 1-855-465-7113

**Special Needs Assistance for Seniors**
Phone: Edmonton,
780-427-7876
or toll-free 1-800-642-3853

### Personal Directive

**Advance Healthcare Directive**
*www.advancecareplanning.ca/provincialresources*

**The Office of the Public Guardian**

Phone: Edmonton,
780-427-0017
Calgary, 403-297-3364
Toll-free 310-0000 and ask for one of the above numbers.

## BRITISH COLUMBIA

### Provincial Health Care Insurance

**Medical Services Plan (MSP)**

Phone: Vancouver, 604-683-7151
Toll-free 1-800-663-7100

**Social Assistance**
Phone: 1-800-663-7867

**BC Palliative Care Benefits Program**

Phone: 604-806-8821
or toll-free 1-877-422-4722
e-mail: bchpca@direct.ca

### Supplementary Income programs

**Persons with Disabilities Benefits Ministry of Human Resources**

Phone: 1-800-663-7867

**Last Post Fund**
Phone: 1-800-268-0248

**Special Needs Assistance for Seniors**

Phone: 1-800-663-7867

### Living Wills and Advance Treatment Directives

A booklet entitled *Let Me Decide* (BC Special Edition – ISBN 968801080, Newgrange Press) is available.
Contact: *idecide@sympatico.ca.*

### Legal Services

**Legal Services Society Law Line**

Phone: Vancouver, 604-687-4680 or toll free 1-800-565-5297.

### Funeral Costs

**Ministry assistance with funeral costs**
contact the local Employment and Assistance Centre.

Phone: Vancouver,
604-660-2421
Victoria, 250-387-6121
Toll-free 1-800-663-7867.

**Public Guardian and Trustee of BC Adult Guardianship project**

Phone: 604-660-4444
Website: *www.trustee.bc.ca*

## MANITOBA

### Provincial Health Care Insurance

**Manitoba Health**

Phone: 204-786-7101
or toll free 1-800-392-1207

T.D.D. (hearing impaired)
call 1-204-774-8618

### Social Assistance

**Manitoba Health, Human Resources**

Phone: 204-948-4000 or
toll free 1-800-563-8793

**Palliative Care Drug Program**
Phone: 204-786-7141

### Supplementary Income Programs for Handicapped Persons

**Employment and Income Assistance**
Phone: 204-945-4437

**Last Post Fund**
Phone: 204-233-3073
or toll-free 1-800-465-7113

### Special Needs Assistance For Seniors

**Seniors Directorate**
Phone: 204-945-6565

**Health Care Directive**
**Seniors Information Line**Phone:
Winnipeg, 204-945-6565 or
toll free 1-800-665-6565

**Office Of The Public Trustee**

Phone: Winnipeg, 204-945-2700
or toll free 1-800-282-
8069, Ext. 2700

## HEALTH LINKS

**(Social and Health Issues)**
Provides information on any health related questions

Phone: 204-788-8200 or
toll free 1-888-315-9257

## NEW BRUNSWICK

### Provincial Health Care Insurance

**Medicare**
Phone: 1-888-762-8600

### Social Assistance

**Family and Community Services – Human Resources Development**
Phone: 1-800-442-9799

**Palliative Care Drug Coverage Special Authorization for Drug Coverage**
Phone: 1-800-332-3692

### Supplementary Income Programs for Handicapped Persons

**See Social Assistance**
**Last Post Fund**
Phone: Saint John, 506-658-9707
or toll-free 1-800-465-7113

### Personal Directive

**Advance Healthcare Directive**
*www.advancecareplanning.ca/provincialresources*

**Power of Attorney for Personal Care**
Phone: 506-453-5369

## NEWFOUNDLAND

### Provincial Health Care Insurance

**Medical Care Plan (MCP)** Phone: 1-800-563-1557

**Red Cross Healthcare Equipment Loans Program**
Phone: 709-758-8414

**Last Post Fund**

Phone: 709-579-4288 or toll-free 1-800-465-7113

**Veteran's Affairs**
Phone: English: 1-866-522-2122 French: 1-866-522-2022

### Personal Directive

**Advance Healthcare Directive**
*www.advancecareplanning.ca/provincialresources*

## NOVA SCOTIA

### Social Assistance

**Employment Support and Income Assistance – Human Resources**
Toll-free 1-877-424-1177

### Palliative Care Drug Coverage

**Nova Scotia Senior's Pharmacare Program**
Phone: 902-429-6565
or toll-free 1-800-544-6191

**Medical Services Insurance (MSI)**
1-800-563-8880
Website: *novascotia.ca/DHW/*

### Supplementary Income Programs for Handicapped Persons

**Disabled Persons Commission**
Phone: 902-424-8280
or toll-free 1-800-277-9914

**Last Post Fund**

Phone: 902-455-5283
or toll-free 1-800-465-7113

### Special Needs Assistance for Seniors

**Senior Citizen's Secretariat Senior Information Line**
Phone: 902-424-0065
or toll-free 1-800-670-0065
e-mail: *SCS@gov.ns.ca*

## ONTARIO

**Provincial Health Care Insurance Government Income Security Program**

Phone: 1-800-277-9914

### Social Assistance

**Community and Social Services (Ontario Ministry of) – Ontario Social Assistance**

Toll-free 1-800-265-3790

### Palliative Care Drug Coverage

**Ministry of Health and Long-Term Care, Drug Programs Branch**
Phone: 416-327-8109

**Last Post Fund**

Toll-free 1-800-465-7113

### Special Needs Assistance for Seniors

**Ministry of Health & Long-Term Care, Assistance Services Programs**
Phone: 416-327-8804

### Personal Directive

**Advance Healthcare Directive**
*www.advancecareplanning.ca/provincialresources*

**Ministry of Health & Long Term Care**

Phone: 1-800-268-1154
*Website: www.health.gov.on.ca*

**Free Guide to Advance Care Planning**
Phone: 1-888-910-1999
*Website: www.seniors.gov.on.ca/en/advancedcare/*

## PRINCE EDWARD ISLAND

### Provincial Health Care Insurance

**Medicare**
Phone: 902-838-0900
or toll-free 1-800-321-5492

### Health Information

**Health Information Resource Centre**
Phone: 902-368-6526

**Island Helpline:** 1-800-218-2885

### Provincial Drug Cost Assistance Program

**Provincial Pharmacy**
Phone: 902-368-4947
or toll-free 1-877-577-3737

### Provincial Palliative Care Program

**Program Coordinator**
Phone: (902) 368-6130

**PEI Council of People with Disabilities**
Phone: 902-892-9149

**Last Post Fund**
Phone: 1-800-465-7113

**PEI Branch**
Phone: 1-800-561-0505

**Seniors Drug Cost Assistance Program**

Phone: 1-877-577-3737

**PEI Senior Citizens' Federation Inc.**

Phone: 902-368-9008
e-mail: *peiscf@pei.aibn.com*

## QUEBEC

- In Quebec province, all medications needed for terminal care are covered by public or private insurance.
- Everyone in Quebec province who needs help for home palliative care services is referred to the local CSSS (Centre de santé et de services sociaux). The CSSSs are responsible for the Home Care Services in the province. The services may be slightly different from one locality to another one, but they all have Home Care Services.
- CSSSs are also responsible for all Social Services and Assistance. They will direct anyone who needs help to the correct services.

**Association des CLSC et des CHSLD du Québec (CSSS) Association des CSSS et des CHSLD du Québec**

White pages of local telephone book or, Phone: 514-931-1448

Website: *sante.gouv.qc.ca/systeme-sante-en-bref/csss/*

### Provincial Health Insurance

**Régie de l'assurance-maladie du Québec (RAMQ)**

Phone: Montreal, 514-864-3411
Quebec City, 418-646-4636
Toll-free 1-800-561-9749

*Website: www.ramq.gouv.qc.ca.*

### Social Assistance

**Ministère de l'emploi et de la solidarité sociale**
Phone: 1-888-643-4721

### Supplementary Income Programs for Handicapped Persons

**Local CLSC office (see above)**

### Special Needs Assistance for Seniors

**Local CLSC office (see above)**

### Death Benefit

**Ministère de l'emploi et de la solidarité sociale**

Phone: 1-888-643-4721

**Last Post Fund**

Phone: 514-866-2888
or toll-free 1-800-465-7113

**Personal Directive Mandate in Case of Incapacity Le Curateur public**

Phone: 1-800-363-9020
Website: *www.curateur.gouv.qc.ca*

**Legal Affairs Communication-Québec**

Phone: 1-877-644-4545
e-mail: *communication-québec@mrci.gouv.qc.ca*

Website: *www.gouv.qc.ca*

**Registry of Death Directeur de l'état civil**

Phone: 1-800-567-3900
e-mail: *etatcivil@dec.gouv.qc.cq*
Website: *www.etatcivil.gouv.qc.ca*

**Advance Healthcare Directive**
*www.advancecareplanning.ca/provincialresources*

## SASKATCHEWAN

### Provincial Health Care Insurance

**Saskatchewan Health**

Phone: 306-787-3124 or
toll-free 1 800-667-7581

### Social Assistance

**Saskatchewan Community Resources and Employment**

Toll Free: 1-877-696-7546

### Palliative Care Drug Coverage

**Saskatchewan Health Drug Plan & Extended Benefits Branch Saskatchewan**

Phone: 306-787-3420
Email: *dpebweb@health.gov.sk.ca*

### Supplementary Income Programs for Handicapped Persons

**Saskatchewan Senior Citizens Provincial Council**
Phone: 306-787-7432

**Last Post Fund**
Phone: 306-975-6045
or toll-free 1-800-465-7113

**Special Needs Assistance for Seniors Ministry of Social Services Seniors' Secretariat**
Phone: 1-800-667-7161

**Saskatchewan Senior Citizens Provincial Council**
Phone: 306-787-7432

### Personal Directive

**The Health Care Directives and Substitute Health Care Decision Makers Act**

Phone: 306-787-6281
*www.advancecareplanning.ca/provincialresources*

## YUKON

### Territorial Health Care Insurance

**Yukon Health Care Insurance Services**

Phone: 867-667-5209
or 1-800-661-0408
e-mail: hss@gov.yk.ca

### Social Assistance

**Health and Social Services**
**Government of Yukon**

Phone: 867-667-3673 or toll-free 1-800-661-0408
e-mail: hss@gov.yk.ca

### Palliative Care Drug Coverage

**Pharmacare**
Phone: 867-667-5403

### Supplementary Income Programs for Handicapped Persons

**Insured Services**
**Health and Social Services**
**Government of Yukon**

Phone: 867-667-5209
or toll-free 1-800-661-0408, local 5209
e-mail: hss@gov.yk.ca

**Last Post Fund**
**British Columbia Branch**
Phone: 1-800-268-0248
e-mail: lastpost@telus.net

### Special Needs Assistance for Seniors

**Extended Healthcare Benefits for Seniors**
Phone: 867-667-5403
or 1-800-661-0408
e-mail: hss@gov.yk.ca

## NWT

**Territorial Health Care Insurance:** 1-800-661-0830

**Social Assistance:** 1-800-661-0830

**Palliative Care Drug Coverage:** 1-800-661-0830

Web Site: *www.hss.gov.nt.ca/*

## NUNAVUT

**Territorial Health Care Insurance:**
867-979-5700

**Social Assistance:**
867-979-5700

**Palliative Care Drug Coverage:**
867-979-5700
Web Site: *www.gov.nu.ca/health*

## APPENDIX VII
# COMPASSIONATE CARE PROGRAM

■

In January 2004, the federal government launched the Compassionate Care Benefit Program under the Employment Insurance Program. Details of the Compassionate Care Program are as follows.

- The new provisions will pay up to six weeks of special benefits to claimants who provide care or support to a gravely ill family member.
- Claimants have access to this new EI special benefit if they have 600 hours of insurable employment in their qualifying period. (The same rules are used as for existing EI special benefits programs such as sickness, maternity and paternal).
- Family members are defined as a spouse or common-law partner, a parent, a spouse or common-law partner of a parent, a child, or a child of the spouse or common-law partner.
- The new provision requires a waiting period, but when eligible family members share the benefits the waiting period may be deferred for all but one family member.
- Claimants need to obtain a medical certificate from a doctor indicating that the family member is gravely ill with a significant risk of death in the next 26 weeks (six months), and that there is a need for one or more family members to provide the ill family member with care or support.
- The government has also made related amendments to the Canada Labour Code to establish an entitlement to a period of leave of up to eight weeks duration with job protection within a 26-week period, for the purpose of providing compassionate care to a family member. This means an employee cannot be fired for asking for or taking up to eight weeks leave to provide compassionate care for a family member.

In 2012, the Federal Employment Insurance Program (EI) announced plans to extend the benefit for up to 35 weeks for parental caregivers of critically ill children under the age of 18. "Critically ill" defined as a life-threatening illness or injury which can include various acute phases of illness or injury where continued parental care or support is required.

**Service Canada Website:s**

*www.servicecanada.gc.ca/eng/ei/types/compassionate_care.shtml*

Information is also available from the Employment Insurance office in your community.

## APPENDIX VIII

# PLANNING AHEAD FOR THE FUNERAL

■

Though often many find this difficult to think about and do, those who have discussed and prepared the funeral ahead of time have found it a great help and relief to them and their family once it is done. Prearranging a funeral allows time to learn the options available, gather a comparison of goods and services provided by a variety of sources, and determine preferences. Details such as the type of service (i.e., traditional, cremation, direct disposition), music, clergy, casket and donations can be discussed and decided upon as well.

Discussion can also take place on ways to personalize the funeral with traditional tributes including those people they wish to speak or deliver a eulogy, and poems or songs to be used. Many new innovations exist to memorialize in ways that provide great comfort to loved ones, including video tributes and special services. The funeral home can review the many options available.

Whatever decision is made can be recorded and kept on file at the funeral home – with copies for family members and executor. Make sure pertinent family members and the executor are aware of the prearrangements made and know where to go at the time of need. It is not a good idea to just record funeral wishes in a will, as the will may not be accessed in a timely manner and generally does not provide the level of detail that the funeral home prearrangement records would contain.

The two main benefits of prearranging a funeral are that it relieves the family from the stress and pressure of having to make critical and highly personal decisions at the actual difficult time of loss, and that it can save an estate thousands of dollars.

| QUESTIONS THAT ARE OFTEN ASKED... | RESPONSES MAY INCLUDE: |
|---|---|
| **How much will it cost and how long for the visit to prearrange a funeral?** | It shouldn't cost a penny and only takes about an hour to complete. Some funeral homes will even arrange for someone to meet the person who is unable to go to the funeral home. |

| | |
|---|---|
| **What information is needed?** | Aside from standard vital statistics, you should be able to give as much or as little information and make as many or few decisions as you wish. However, the more information you provide now, the fewer unanswered questions there will be later. |
| **At the end of the prearrangement meeting, will a cost quote be provided?** | A quote to prepay the funeral service should be provided without obligation. You can comparison shop. However, if you have a good relationship with a particular funeral home, that is often more important than cost. |
| **What if we change our minds about what is wanted?** | You should be allowed to update or change arrangements at any time and as many times as you wish. Keep in mind that changes may alter the price quoted. |
| **Can the cost be locked into today's prices?** | Most funeral homes offer this option if you prepay your arrangements. Changes can still be made in the future. However, the change may or may not be included in the locked in price. |
| **What options are available to prepay a funeral?** | Lump sum and time-pay (usually one to 10 years) options are usually offered. Often, the quicker the payment, the bigger the discount. |
| **Can a refund be obtained if there is a cancellation or change of the prearrangement contract?** | Find out if full or partial refunds are offered and whether there are any holdbacks or penalty fees. |

Adapted from *Taking Care of Loved Ones Affairs* (2012) Ottawa, Ontario: Inevitable Exodus Inc.

# APPENDIX IX
# HISTORY OF *A CAREGIVER'S GUIDE*

■

Since 2000 the Order of St. Lazarus in Canada has enabled the distribution of more than 300,000 copies of *A Caregiver's Guide* to caregivers across Canada at no cost to the recipients. Canadian editions have been published in English, French, Traditional Chinese Characters and two Inuit languages End-of-life care organizations in Portugal, Australia, China, Japan and Slovenia have also translated and distributed the book.

The original edition was a joint project of the Edmonton and Calgary Commanderies of the Order of St. Lazarus and the Palliative Care Association of Alberta. It is the result of contributions and review from family caregivers and numerous Albertan palliative care professionals in the fields of nursing, medicine, social work, pharmacy, nutrition, physiotherapy, occupational therapy and pastoral counseling. It was designed to assist family caregivers by complementing the guidance and assistance they receive from palliative care and home care professionals.

Over a 12-month period beginning in 1998, suggestions for the design, format and content of *A Caregiver's Guide* were received from palliative care workers across the province of Alberta. A team of experienced palliative care professionals and health educators reviewed, compiled and wrote *A Caregiver's Guide* based on this input. After extensive internal review, draft copies were sent to both palliative care professionals and lay caregivers on two occasions. The final product resulted from the careful consideration of their responses.

*A Caregiver's Guide* soon became a mainstay of end-of life care in Alberta and many requests for the book were received from organizations in other Canadian provinces. Encouraged by Senator Sharon Carstairs (then Minister with special responsibility for palliative care, now retired) the Order of St. Lazarus committed to developing a national edition of *A Caregiver's Guide*. The Canadian Hospice Palliative Care association agreed to endorse this edition and enable distribution of it to end-of-life care organizations and programs across Canada.

This revised edition will continue to serve Canadian caregivers for years to come.

**Acknowledgements from the 2000 Edition**

We also wish to thank and recognize the following individuals, companies and organizations, all of whom played an essential role in the development of the 2000 edition of *A Caregiver's Guide*:

The contributors and reviewers are far too numerous to mention, but for the most part were involved with either supporting or providing palliative care services through Alberta's health regions. Karen Macmillan and Jacquie Peden compiled the first draft as nurse consultants for the Capital Health (Edmonton) Regional Palliative Care Program. Jane Hopkinson provided excellent editorial review and coordination.

For their generous financial support without which publication and distribution of *A Caregiver's Guide* would not have been possible:

- Jack and Shirley Singer.
- United Active Living.
- The Alberta Cancer Foundation.
- The Capital Health Authority Regional Palliative Care Program and its medical, nursing and other staff members who so generously supported and contributed to this project.
- Family Health magazine, and especially Cathy Berry, administrative assistant, who throughout the development of this project provided much needed administrative and logistical support, co-ordination of editorial copy flow and other production support.
- The director and members of the Palliative Care Association of Alberta who actively contributed to the planning and review of *A Caregiver's Guide*.
- The members of the Calgary and Edmonton Commanderies of the Order of St. Lazarus who, in so many ways, supported the publication of this book.
- The valuable contributions from Rob Weideman with the design, layout and illustration of *A Caregiver's Guide*.

The publishers would especially like to thank the following individuals and organizations for their contributions to the editorial content:

- The staff of McGill University Health Centre, Palliative Care Program, especially Nathalie Aubin and Martin Lavergne, Montreal, PQ
- Donalda Carson, Hospice Prince George, Prince George, BC
- Sharon Baxter, Executive Director and Greg Adams, Administrative Co-ordinator, Canadian Hospice Palliative Care Association

We also wish to recognize those numerous palliative care and home care professionals whose mission is to help their fellow Albertans through this difficult time of life.

- Dennie Hycha, President, Palliative Care Association of Alberta
- Robert Clarke, Commander, Edmonton, The Order of St. Lazarus

### Acknowledgements from the 2004 Edition

A revised, national edition was reviewed by members of the original writing team as well as palliative care professionals from across Canada.

We wish to acknowledge the following contributions which have greatly assisted the publication and distribution of the 2004 revised national edition of *A Caregiver's Guide*:

**For their generous financial support:**

- Great West Life, London Life and Canada Life.
- Charles R. Vint Estate.
- Alberta Cancer Foundation.
- Jackman Foundation.
- Department of Canadian Heritage, Assistance for Translation Program.
- Pallium Network.
- Grant James Gehlsen, CLJ.
- Edmonton Commandery, Order of St. Lazarus.
- Montreal Commandery, Order of St. Lazarus.

**For editorial and administrative support:**

- The members and staff of Canadian Hospice Palliative Care Association, and the Palliative Care Association of Alberta made numerous contributions to this revised national edition, especially its distribution.
- Joni Millar and Jillian Millar Drysdale of Tilt Creative, Jan Crouch of *Family Health* Magazine and Jean Matheson of the Order of St. Lazarus, contributed greatly to the production and administration.
- The enthusiastic support of the Honourable Senator (retired) Sharon Carstairs was instrumental in encouraging the publishers to proceed with this edition.
- Gael Page, President.
- Sharon Baxter, Executive Director.
  Canadian Hospice Palliative Care Association
- Robert W. Clarke, KCLJ, Chairman, Medical Commission
- Robert H. Vandewater, GCLJ, Grand Prior., The Order of St. Lazarus

## APPENDIX X
# THE MILITARY AND HOSPITALLER ORDER OF ST. LAZARUS OF JERUSALEM

*In 2011, wildfires swept through Slave Lake, Alberta. The disaster destroyed 40% of the town leaving men, women, and children homeless. Recognizing the trauma of the injured children, the Order of St. Lazarus sent 75 teddy bears for comfort. The response was overwhelming. Today some of these bears are still displayed in rebuilt store windows in tribute to the Order's caring.*

The Order of St. Lazarus's commitment to responding compassionately to immediate needs reaches back to the 11th century. Much has changed in 900 years, but people in need continue to require compassion, comfort and care.

The Order's story begins in 1099 as the knights and soldiers of the First Crusade entered Jerusalem. The sick and wounded crowded the city, but those suffering from leprosy were segregated outside the walls in an ancient leper hospice. One French monk, assisted by crusaders who had themselves contracted the disease, took on the onerous challenge of caring for all lepers, regardless of their religion.

Following the end of the Crusades, the knights and monks of St. Lazarus became responsible for operating leprosy hospitals (Lazar Houses) throughout Europe in countries like England, Scotland, and France.

The Order arrived in Canada (New France) in 1599 when Henri IV appointed the Grand Master of the Order as the Lieutenant General of New France. With the fall of New France in 1763 the Order ceased its activities in North America. It returned to Canada in 1962 when the Honourable J. Keiller MacKay, the Lieutenant Governor of Ontario, arranged for the investiture of twenty Knights, Dames and Commanders in Toronto and was himself installed as the first Grand Bailiff.

Over the past 50 years, the Grand Priory in Canada has grown to approximately 400 members in thirteen local branches (known as Commanderies or Delegations) stretching from St. John's to Victoria. A bilingual, registered charitable organization, it welcomes women and men into its ranks. Globally, the Order maintains its ancient, Christian heritage and original mandate to assist those suffering from leprosy.

The Order in Canada has adopted hospice/palliative care as a primary mission. For the most part, the Order collaborates with other Hospice/Palliative Care organizations within the various commandery areas by lending its resources, both human and financial.

One example is the publication of *A Caregiver's Guide*. The Alberta commanderies worked closely with the provincial palliative care community to create this much-needed resource. Since the initial publication in 2000, the Order has sponsored the national printing and distribution of more than 275,000 copies in English, French, two Inuit languages, and Traditional Chinese Characters. The book is now considered one of the go-to resources for organizations and individuals caring for patients and loved ones. Its use has been adopted internationally with translated editions published in Portugal, Australia, China, and Japan.

Putting our mandate into practice also includes a personal touch. In Ontario, when a local hospital could not find the funds to spruce up its palliative care room, a member personally painted the space. It had been neglected for ten years. The fresh paint and evidence of care greatly alleviated the distress of families sitting through their loved ones' final days.

Another program makes teddy bears available to palliative patients of all ages. In one instance, a man who was nearing his end was fearful and agitated. He rejected all his wife's attempts to comfort him until he was given a St. Lazarus teddy bear. Cuddling the bear calmed him and he died peacefully with his wife holding his other hand. She now treasures this bear and the role it played near the end of her husband's life.

These are but a few examples of how the Order of St. Lazarus in Canada fulfills its ancient mission of caring for people in need. The Order is also committed to honouring its Christian heritage.

In Canada, the Order's support is committed to furthering ecumenism in its broadest sense. To this end it established scholarships and study bursaries for students pursuing ecumenical studies in fifteen universities and seminaries across the country.

Service to people of all faiths and cultures permeates the day-to-day activities of the Order in Canada. When asked what the Order of St. Lazarus stands for, our response is:

*"We are dedicated to the service of the sick and dying of all faiths, to unity amongst Christians and the eradication of leprosy."*

**Further information about the Order of St. Lazarus and the work we do can be found at *www.stlazarus.ca*.**

* * *

Following are examples of palliative care programs and projects with which the Order of St. Lazarus has been involved:

### Acadia Commadery

Colchester East Hants Hospice Society

Bobby's Hospice – Hospice Greater Saint John

The Hospice Society of Greater Halifax

Hospice Greater Moncton

Hospice Miramichi

New Brunswick Hospice Palliative Care Association

### Arctic Delegation

Cooperation with Avens Society and Yellowknife Association for Concerned Citizens

Stanton Territorial Hospital

Elders Traditional Medicine Advisory Committee

Development of a video version of *A Caregiver's Guide* for the Aboriginal community

Community Health Centers in the Northwest Territories and Nunavut

Hospice Yukon

### British Columbia Delegation

Palliative Care Unit, Royal Jubilee Hospital Victoria Hospice Society

### Calgary Commandery

Hospice Calgary

St. Michael's, Lethbridge

Foothills Country Hospice

Alberta Hospice Palliative Care Association

Red Deer Hospice

High River District Health Care Foundation

St. Lazarus "Teddy Bear" program for palliative care

### Edmonton Commandery

Kairos House hospice for men and women with HIV/AIDS

Red Deer Hospice

Pilgrim's Hospice

Alberta Hospice Palliative Care Association

Edmonton Regional Palliative Care Program

Palliative Care Bursary at MacEwan University

Palliative Care chairs and related furnishings at Kipnes Centre, Norwood Hospice and Royal Alexandra, Wetaskiwin, Good Samaritan and St. Joseph's hospitals

Concept and editorial development of *A Caregiver's Guide*

### Manitoba Delegation

Hospice Manitoba

Grace Hospice

Saint Boniface Palliative Care

### Montreal Commandery

The West Island Hospice

SSPAD - Montreal and Laval

Nova West Island (Old VON)

Montreal General Hospital - Palliative Care Unit

### Newfoundland and Labrador Delegation

Supports various provincial palliative care initiatives

### Ottawa Commandery

Hospice at May Court

Perley & Rideau Veteran's Foundation

Hospice at the Union Mission

Ottawa Hospice Foundation

Algonquin College

Hospice Renfrew

Outcare Foundation

### Québec Commandery

Fondation l'aube Nouvelle (soins palliatifs)

Fondation CPSQ (Centre de prévention du suicide)

Fondation Marc-André Jacques (soins palliatifs)

Abbé Denis Cadrin (œuvres paroissiales)

Paroisse St-Rédempteur (étudiants en soins palliatifs)

Fondation Equilibrium psychologique

Fondation C.E.G.E.P. La Pocatière ( étudiants en soins palliatifs)

Fondation C.E.G.E.P. Matane (étudiants en soins palliatifs)

Fondations : Hôpital Laval, Enfant-Jésus, St-François d'Assise

Centre de réadaptation Hôpital Laval

La Fondation Gilles-Kègle

**Thunder Bay Commandery**

Regional Palliative Care programs and initiatives

Support to graduates of the Canadian Nurse Association Certification in Hospice Palliative Care

St. Lazarus "Teddy Bear" program for palliative care

Sponsorship of speakers in palliative care to the Thunder Bay Council of Clergy

**Western Ontario Commandery**

Hospice Waterloo

Hospice London

South Huron Regional Health Centre

Collaboration with St. John Ambulance in the Home Caregiver Support Program

**Toronto Commandery**

Toronto Commandery Hospice Foundation

Dorothy Ley Hospice

Emily's House

Hospice Peterborough

Muskoka Hospice

McDermott House Canada

Hill House Hospice

Hospice Palliative Care Ontario

HPCO "Embracing Diversity" Conference

Hospice King-Aurora

Humber College Palliative Care Conference

Palliative Care Information Centre

Rose Cherry's Home

The Palliative Care Foundation

Toronto Grace Health Centre Palliative Care

Trinity Home Hospice

The National Grand Priory of the Order of St. Lazarus of Jerusalem in Canada co-ordinates all aspects of publishing *A Caregiver's Guide* and in part funded the development of both this 2014 revised edition and the 2004 edition which it replaces. To date, more than 300,000 copies have been distributed to Canadians from coast to coast to coast and to numerous international stakeholders. *A Caregiver's Guide* was originally developed in 2000 by the Edmonton and Calgary commanderies of the Order of St. Lazarus. The Edmonton, Calgary and Western Ontario commanderies of the Order funded the distribution of more than 24,000 copies of the original edition to Canadians caring for loved ones in their communities. *A Caregiver's Guide* has been now translated into nine languages with and published internationally in Australia, Portugal, China and Japan; additional international editions are planned for 2014 and beyond.

# APPENDIX XI
# CANADIAN HOSPICE PALLIATIVE CARE ASSOCIATION

■

The Canadian Hospice Palliative Care Association (CHPCA) is the national voice for hospice palliative care in Canada. It is a bilingual, national charitable non-profit association whose mission is the pursuit of excellence in care for persons approaching death so that the burdens of suffering, loneliness and grief are lessened.

The CHPCA strives to achieve its mission through:

- collaboration and representation;
- increased awareness, knowledge and skills related to hospice palliative care of the public, health care providers and volunteers;
- development of national norms of practice for hospice palliative care in Canada;
- support of research on hospice palliative care;
- advocacy for improved hospice palliative care policy, resource allocation and supports for caregivers.

Since its inception in 1993 the CHPCA has been working in close partnership with the 11 provincial hospice palliative care associations (see the resource section for provincial contact information) and with other national organizations such as the Quality End-of-Life Care Coalition.

The CHPCA will continue to move forward with the goal of ensuring that all Canadians, regardless of where they may live, have equal access to quality hospice palliative care services for themselves and their family.

## THE ORIGINS OF HOSPICE PALLIATIVE CARE

Dame Cicely Saunders first conceived of the modern hospice movement in the United Kingdom in the mid-1960s to care for the dying.[1] Balfour Mount coined the term palliative care (from the Latin palliare = to cloak or cover[2]) in 1975 so that one term would be acceptable in both English and French as he brought the movement to Canada.

Both hospice and palliative care movements have flourished in Canada and internationally. Palliative care programs developed primarily within larger health care institutions, while hospice care developed within the community as free-standing, primarily volunteer programs. Over time, these programs gradually evolved from individual, grassroots efforts to a cohesive movement that aims to relieve suffering and improve quality of life for those who are living with, or dying from, an illness.

To recognize the convergence of hospice and palliative care and their common norms of practice into one movement, the term hospice palliative care was coined. While hospice palliative care is the nationally accepted term to describe care aimed at relieving suffering and improving quality of life, individual organizations may continue to use hospice, palliative care, or another similarly acceptable term to describe their organizations and the services they are providing.

1 *Saunders C. A personal therapeutic journey. BMJ 1996; 313(7072): 1599-601.*

2 *Little W, Fowler HW, Coulson J. The Shorter Oxford English Dictionary (Onions CT (ed.) Toronto, Ontario: Oxford University Press*

## PROVINCIAL ASSOCIATIONS

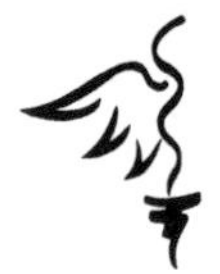

**Canadian Hospice Palliative Care Association**
**Association canadienne de soins palliatifs**

Saint Vincent Hospital, Annex D,
60 Cambridge Street North
Ottawa, Ontario K1R 7A5

*Telephone:* (613) 241-3663
or (800) 668-2785
*Fax:* (613) 241-3986

*info@chpca.net* | *www.chpca.net*

AHPCA

**Alberta Hospice Palliative Care Association**

1245 - 70 Avenue SE
Calgary, AB T2H 2X8

*Telephone:* (403) 206-9938
*Fax:* (403) 206-9958

*director@ahpca.ca* | *www.ahpca.ca*

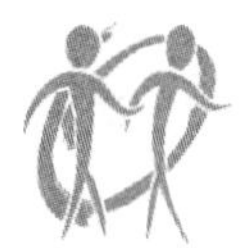

**Réseau de soins palliatifs du Québec (AQSP)**

Case postale 361, Succursale
Saint-Charles, Kirkland,
Quebec H9H 0A5

*Telephone:* (514) 826-9400

*info@aqsp.org* | *www.aqsp.org*

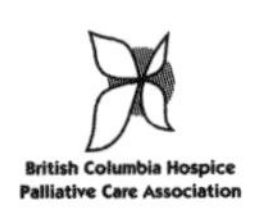


**British Columbia Hospice Palliative Care Association**

Suite 1100-1200, West 73rd Ave.
Vancouver B.C. V6P 6G5

*Telephone:* 1.877.422.4722

*office@bchpca.org* | *www.bchpca.org*

HOSPICE

### Hospice Palliative Care Ontario

2 Carlton Street, Suite 707,
Toronto ON
M5B 1J3

*Telephone:* (416) 304-1477
*Toll-free:* (800) 349-3111
*Fax:* (416) 304-1479

*info@hpco.ca* | *www.hpco.ca*

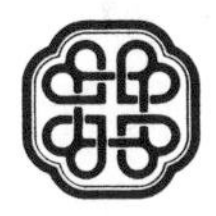

### Hospice & Palliative Care Manitoba

2109 Portage Avenue,
Winnipeg MB R3J 0L3

*Telephone:* (204) 889-8525
*Toll-free:* (800) 539-0295
(Manitoba only)

*info@manitobahospice.mb.ca* | *www.manitobahospice.ca*

### Hospice Palliative Care Association of PEI

5 Brighton Road,
Charlottetown, PEI, C1A 8T6

*Telephone:* 902-368-4498
*Fax:* 902-368-4095

*hpca@hospicepei.ca* | *www.hospicepei.ca*

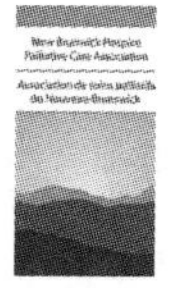

### New Brunswick Hospice Palliative Care Association

PO Box 406,
Simon Larouche Pavillion
165 Hebert Blvd.,
Edmundston, NB E3V 2S8

*Telephone:* (506) 623-6383
*Fax:* (506) 454-1650

*info@nbhpca-aspnb.ca* | *www.nbhpca-aspnb.ca*

### Newfoundland and Labrador Palliative Care Association

PO Box 39023, 390 Topsail Road
St. John's, NL A1E 5Y7

*Telephone:* 709-786-7395
*Fax:* (709) 777-8635

*exec@nlpalliativecareassociation.com* | *nlpalliativecareassociation.com*

Nova Scotia Hospice Palliative Care Association

### Nova Scotia Hospice Palliative Care Association

PO Box 103
Lakeside, Nova Scotia B3T 1M6

*Telephone:* 1 (902) 818-9139

*info@nshpca.ca* | *www.nshpca.ca*

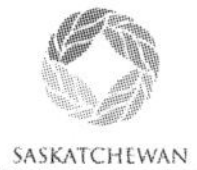
SASKATCHEWAN HOSPICE PALLIATIVE CARE ASSOCIATION INC.

### Saskatchewan Hospice Palliative Care Association

Box 37053
Regina, Saskatchewan, S4S 7K3

*Telephone:* (306) 522-3232

*info@saskpalliativecare.org* | *www.saskpalliativecare.org*

# INDEX

■

## A

Adapting your home **25**
Addiction **76**
Analgesic, explained **72**
Analgesic ladder **73**
Anticipatory grief **131**
Appetite, decreasing **52**

## B

Bathing **30**
Bathroom, helping to use **48**
Bed bath **31**
Bedpans **50**
Books to help grieving children **138**
Bowel and bladder problems
- constipation **87**
- diarrhea **89**
- incontinence **86**

## C

Canadian Hospice Palliative Care Association **173**
- provincial associations **174**

Caregiver "burnout" **14**
Caring for yourself
- coping skills **12**
- managing your emotions **12**
- what you can do **11**

Cold treatments, comfort from **104**
Commodes **49**
Communication
- guidelines for conversation **19**
- ideas to help **18**
- with children **21**
- with family **20**
- with the healthcare team **22**
- with visitors **23**

Compassionate Care Program **162**
Complementary care
- cold treatments **104**
- distraction **103**
- heat treatments **106**
- herbal remedies **108**
- imagery **102**
- relaxation breathing **102**
- relaxation techniques **101**
- vibration massage **103**

Confusion **99**
- comfort and care **100**
- hallucination **99**

Constipation **87**
- comfort and care **88**
- enemas **89**
- explained **87**

Contact names and numbers **4**

## D

Death
- advance planning of final arrangements **119**
- arrangements after **119**
- benefits **123**
- comfort, yourself and loved ones **118**
- decisions after **119**
- funeral / memorial service **120**
- if death happens at home **117**
- necessary personal information **121**
- places to notify **122**
- signs of approach **116**

Diarrhea **89**
- comfort and care **90**
- foods to avoid **90**

Distraction **103**

Dyspnea **91**
- comfort and care **91**
- oygen therapy **93**

## E

Eating
- giving help with **54**
- liquid feedings **59**
- nutritional supplement recipes **58**
- reduced fluid intake **55**

Edema (swelling) **97**

## F

Final thoughts **131**

Financial aid
- associations, lodges and unions **148**
- Canada Customs and Revenue Agency **148**
- Canada / Quebec pension plan **146**
- Canadian Cancer Society and Fondation québecoise du cancer **148**
- employment insurance **147**
- guaranteed income supplement **146**
- Last Post Fund **148**
- life insurance **147**
- old age security **146**
- palliative care drug coverage **147**
- private insurance and supplementary health care plans **147**
- supplementary income programs for handicapped persons **148**
- Veterans Affairs (DVA) **147**

Fluid intake, reduced **55**

Food and fluid changes
- commercial food supplements **51**
- food supplements, homemade **52**
- nutritional supplements **51**

Funeral, planning ahead **163**

## G


Grief 125
- books for children 138
- children and 127
- emotional effect 126
- how long grief lasts 130
- mental effect 126
- physical affect 126
- social effect 127
- spiritual affect 127
- taking care of yourself 128
- what you need to know 125


## H


Heat treatments 106
Herbal remedies 108
History of A Caregiver's Guide 165
Home care services 17
Home medication schedule 151
Hospice palliative care 3


## I


Incontinence 86
Infection control 28
Insomnia 96
Internet resources 139


## L


Legal affairs
- enduring power of attorney 149
- guardianship 149
- mandate in case of incapacity (Quebec only) 150
- old age security trusteeship (limited power of attorney) 150
- personal directive (living will) 150
- trusteeship 149

Life, last days
- changing levels of awareness 114
- withdrawal 114


## M


Vibration Massage 103
Medications 60
- by mouth 63
- by suppository 64
- giving medication 61
- non-opioid pain medications 74
- opioid pain medicines 73
- subcutaneous 66
- transdermal 65

Military and Hospitaller Order of St. Lazarus of Jerusalem 168
Mouth problems
- dry mouth 84
- mouth sores 83
- thrush (oral candidiasis) 82

move to hospice 113

## N

Nausea and vomiting **94**
- comfort and care **94**

Nutritional supplements
- recipes **58**

## O

Opioids
- tolerance **76**
- toxicity **77**

Oxygen therapy **93**

## P

Pain
- assessing pain **70**
- managing with medications **72**
- non-medication pain relief **79**
- TENS (transcutaneous nerve stimulation) **78**

Planning
- dying at home **110**
- practical details **111**

## R

References **142**

Relaxation breathing **102**

Resources that may help **133**

Respite care **13**

## S

Shortness of breath **91**
- oxygen therapy **93**

Side effects
- addiction versus physical dependence **76**
- confusion **76**
- constipation **75**
- drowsiness **75**
- myoclonus **76**
- nausea and vomiting **75**

Skin problems
- bed sores (pressure sores) **81**
- itching **79**

Spiritual needs **23**

St. Lazarus of Jerusalem **168**

Strength, loss of **98**

subcutaneous needle **66**

Support networks **16**
- formal **17**
- informal **16**

Swelling (edema) **97**
- comfort and care **97**

Symptom assessment scale **152**

## T

TENS (transcutaneous nerve stimulation) **78**

Toileting **48**

Toxicity, opioid **77**

## U

Urinals **49**

## W

Wong-Baker pain rating scale, **71**

# NOTES FOR YOU AND YOUR NURSE

■

# NOTES

# WE'D LIKE YOUR HELP

■

We hope that *A Caregiver's Guide* has given you help, support and comfort during a difficult time for your family. Copies of *A Caregiver's Guide* are distributed free of charge to Canadians by more than 500 hospice and palliative care programs through the support of The Military and Hospitaller Order of St. Lazarus of Jerusalem, a registered Canadian charitable organization (Registration Number 11924-5223RR0001). For more information about the Order of St. Lazarus, please refer to (page 168).

The Order would welcome your support to assist in making future editions of *A Caregiver's Guide* available at no cost to Canadians during their time of need. Please help us by returning the coupon below with your donation. Tax receipts will be issued for amounts in excess of $10.00.

Thank you,

The Military and Hospitaller Order of St. Lazarus of Jerusalem

**The Military and Hospitaller Order of St. Lazarus of Jerusalem**
1435 Sandford Fleming Avenue, Suite 100
Ottawa, ON K1G 3H3

I wish to support continued distribution of *A Caregiver's Guide* at no cost to Canadians during their time of need. Enclosed is my donation of :

☐ $10.00 ☐ $25.00 ☐ $50.00 ☐ Other ________

Please issue tax receipt to:

NAME

ADDRESS | PROVINCE | POSTAL CODE

☐ **VISA** ☐ **MASTERCARD** ☐ **CHEQUE (ENCLOSED)**

VISA/MASTERCARD NUMBER | CARDHOLDER NAME | EXPIRY DATE /